Histological Typing of Tumours of the Thymus

W0227824

Springer
Berlin
Heidelberg
New York
Barcelona
Hong Kong
London
Milan
Paris
Singapore
Tokyo

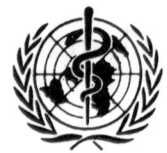 World Health Organization

The series *International Histological Classification of Tumours* consists of the following volumes. The early ones can be ordered through WHO, Distribution and Sales, Avenue Appia, CH-1211 Geneva 27.

 2. Histological typing of breast tumours (1968, second edition 1981)
14. Histological and cytological typing of neoplastic diseases of haematopoietic and lymphoid tissues (1976)
22. Histological typing of prostate tumours (1980)
23. Histological typing of endocrine tumours (1980)

A coded compendium of the International Histological Classification of Tumours (1978).

The following volumes have already appeared in a revised second edition with Springer-Verlag:
Histological Typing of Thyroid Tumours. Hedinger/Williams/Sobin (1988)
Histological Typing of Intestinal Tumours. Jass/Sobin (1989)
Histological Typing of Oesophageal and Gastric Tumours. Watanabe/Jass/Sobin (1990)
Histological Typing of Tumours of the Gallbladder and Extrahepatic Bile Ducts. Albores-Saavedra/Henson/Sobin (1990)
Histological Typing of Tumours of the Upper Respiratory Tract and Ear. Shanmugaratnam/Sobin (1981)
Histological Typing of Salivary Gland Tumours. Seifert (1991)
Histological Typing of Odontogenic Tumours. Kramer/Pindborg/Shear (1992)
Histological Typing of Tumours of the Central Nervous System. Kleihues/Burger/Scheithauer (1993)
Histological Typing of Bone Tumours. Schajowicz (1993)
Histological Typing of Soft Tissue Tumours. Weiss (1994)
Histological Typing of Female Genital Tract Tumours. Scully et al. (1994)
Histological Typing of Tumours of the Liver. Ishak et al. (1994)
Histological Typing of Tumours of the Exocrine Pancreas. Klöppel/Solcia/Longnecker/Capella/Sobin (1996)
Histological Typing of Skin Tumours. Heenan/Elder/Sobin (1996)
Histological Typing of Cancer and Precancer of the Oral Mucosa. Pindborg/Reichart/Smith/van der Waal (1997)
Histological Typing of Kidney Tumours. Mostofi/Davis (1998)
Histological Typing of Testis Tumours. Mostofi/Sesterhenn (1998)
Histological Typing of Tumours of the Eye and Its Adnexa. Campbell (1998)
Histological Typing of Ovarian Tumours. Scully (1999)
Histological Typing of Lung and Pleural Tumours. Travis/Colby/Corrin (1999 third edition)
Histological Typing of Urinary Bladder Tumours. Mostofi/Davis/Sesterhenn (1999)
Histological Typing of Tumours of the Thymus. Rosai (1999)

Histological Typing of Tumours of the Thymus

Juan Rosai

In Collaboration with L.H. Sobin
and Pathologists in 8 Countries

Second Edition

With 70 Colour Figures

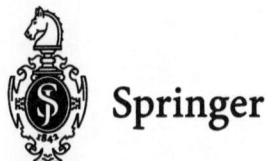 Springer

Juan Rosai, MD
Department of Pathology, Memorial Sloan Kettering Cancer Center
1275 York Avenue, New York, NY 10021, USA

Leslie H. Sobin, MD
WHO Collaborating Center for the International Histological
Classification of Tumours, Armed Forces Institute of Pathology
Washington, DC 20306-6000, USA

ISBN-13:978-3-540-65731-6

Library of Congress Cataloging-in-Publication Data
Rosai, Juan, 1940- Histological typing of tumours of the thymus. - 2nd ed./Juan Rosai; in collabora-
tion with L.H. Sobin and pathologists from 8 countries. p. cm. - (International histological classifica-
tion of tumours) Includes bibliographical references and index.
ISBN-13:978-3-540-65731-6   e-ISBN-13: 978-3-642-60157-6
DOI: 10.1007/978-3-642-60157-6

1. Thymus-Tumours-Classification. 2. Thymus-Tumours-Histopathology. 3. Thymus-Tumours-
Cytodiagnosis. I. Sobin, L.H. II. Title. III. Series: International histological classification of tumours
(Unnumbered)
[DNLM: 1. Thymus Neoplasms-pathology. 2. Thymus Neoplasms-classification. WK 400 R788h
1999] RC280.T55R67 1999 616.99'243-dc21 DNLM/DLC 99-36794

This work is subject to copyright. All rights are reserved, whether the whole or part of the material is
concerned, specifically the rights of translation, reprinting, reuse of illustrations, recitation, broad-
casting, reproduction on microfilm or in any other ways, and storage in data banks. Duplication of this
publication or parts thereof is permitted only under the provisions of the German Copyright Law of
September 9, 1965, in its current version, and permission for use must always be obtained from
Springer-Verlag. Violations are liable for prosecution under the German Copyright Law.

© Springer-Verlag Berlin Heidelberg 1999

The use of general descriptive names, registered names, trademarks, etc. in this publication does not
imply, even in the absence of a specific statement, that such names are exempt from the relevant pro-
tective laws and regulations and therefore free for general use.

Product liability: The publisher cannot guarantee the accuracy of any information about dosage and
application contained in this book. In every individual case the user must check such information by
consulting the relevant literature.

Typesetting: Springer-Verlag, Heidelberg

SPIN: 10718134   24/3135 – 5 4 3 2 1 0 – Printed on acid-free paper.

Participants

Caillaud, Jean-Michel, Dr.
Rhône-Poulenc Rorer, Centre de Recherche,
Vitry-Sur-Seine, France

Elsner, Boris, Dr.
Department of Pathology, Hospital de Clínicas José de San Martín,
Buenos Aires, Argentina

Havlíček, František, Dr.
Department of Pathology, Hospital of the Rudolf and Stefanie,
Prague, Czech Republic

Kuo, Tseng-tong, Dr.
Department of Pathology, Chang Gung Memorial Hospital,
Taipei, Taiwan, Republic of China

Moran, Cesar, Dr.
Department of Pathology, University of Alabama at Birmingham,
Birmingham, AL, USA

Mukai, Kiyoshi, Dr.
Department of Pathology, Tokyo Medical University, Tokyo, Japan

Müller-Hermelink, Hans K., Dr.
Pathologisches Institut, Luitpoldkrankenhaus,
Universität Würzburg, Würzburg, Germany

Palestro, Giorgio, Dr.
Dipartimento di Scienze Biomediche e Oncologia Umana,
Sezione ci Anatomia Patologica, Università Degli Studi di Torino,
Torino, Italy

Rouse, Robert V., Dr.
Department of Pathology, Stanford University Medical Center,
Stanford, CA, USA

Wick, Mark, Dr.
Department of Pathology, University of Virginia Medical Center,
Charlottesville, VA, USA

General Preface to the Series

Among the prerequisites for comparative studies of cancer are international agreement on histological criteria for the classification of cancer types and a standardized nomenclature. At present, pathologists use different terms for the same pathological entity, and, furthermore, the same term is sometimes applied to lesions of different types. An internationally agreed classification of tumours, acceptable alike to physicians, surgeons, radiologists, pathologists, and statisticians, would enable cancer workers in all parts of the world to compare their findings and would facilitate collaboration among them.

In a report published in 1952[1], a subcommittee of the WHO Expert Committee on Health Statistics discussed the general principles that should govern the statistical classification of tumours and agreed that, to ensure the necessary flexibility and ease in coding, three separate classifications were needed according to (1) anatomical site, (2) histological type, and (3) degree of malignancy. A classification according to anatomical site is available in the International Classification of Diseases[2].

In 1956, the WHO Executive Board passed a resolution[3] requesting the Director-General to explore the possibility that WHO might organize centres in various parts of the world and arrange for the collection of human tissues and their histological classification.

The main purpose of such centres would be to develop histological definitions of cancer types and to facilitate the wide adoption of a uniform nomenclature. This resolution was endorsed by the Tenth World Health Assembly in May 1957[4].

---

[1] WHO (1952) WHO Technical Report Series, no. 53. WHO, Geneva, p. 45.

[2] WHO (1977) Manual of the international statistical classification of diseases, injuries, and causes of death, 1975 version. WHO, Geneva.

[3] WHO (1956) WHO Official Records, no. 68, p 14 (resolution EB 17.R40).

[4] WHO (1957) WHO Official Records, no. 79, p. 467 (resolution WHA 10.18).

Since 1958, WHO has established a number of centres concerned with this subject. The result of this endeavor has been the multivolume series, International Histological Classification of Tumours.

Preface to Histological Typing of Tumours of the Thymus

The first WHO series, International Histological Classification of Tumours, did not include a publication on the thymus. Whatever the reason, it is a fact that knowledge of thymic tumours at that time was woefully inadequate. The last two decades have witnessed a renewed interest in this subject on the part of several groups, which has generated a fair amount of new information accompanied by the expected speculations and controversies. The WHO committee which has been assembled to deal with this matter represents pathologists from eight countries and includes many of the individuals who have met on several occasions during the course of the past decade and presented their ongoing proposals and deliberations at international meetings of the International Academy of Pathology in Buenos Aires (1990), Budapest (1996), and Nice (1998), the last in the context of a Seminar on Mediastinal Tumours in which several of the Committee members participated.

It will be appreciated, of course, that the classification reflects the present state of knowledge and that modifications are almost certain to be needed as experience accumulates. Although the present classification has been adopted by the members of the group, it necessarily represents a view from which some pathologists may wish to dissent. Nevertheless, it is hoped that, in the interests of international cooperation, all pathologists will use the classification as proposed. Criticism and suggestions for its improvement will be welcomed; these should be sent to the World Health Organization, 1211 Geneva 27, Switzerland.

The histological classification of thymic tumours, which appears on pp.5-7, contains the morphology code numbers of the International Classification of Diseases for Oncology (ICD-O)[1] and the System-

---

[1] World Health Organization (1990) International classification of diseases for oncology (ICD-O),Geneva.

atized Nomenclature of Medicine (SNOMED)[2]. The publications in the series, *International Histological Classification of Tumours*, are not intended to serve as textbooks, but rather to promote the adoption of a uniform terminology that will facilitate communication among cancer workers. For this reason, literature references have intentionally been omitted and readers should refer to standard works for bibliographies.

[2] College of American Pathologists (1982) Systematized nomenclature of medicine (SNOMED). Chicago, IL.

Contents

Introduction

The term thymoma, formerly used to designate a large variety of histologically unrelated tumours involving the thymus, is now restricted to neoplasms arising from – or differentiating towards – thymic epithelial cells, regardless of the presence and relative number of non-neoplastic lymphocytes. Although in a generic sense all thymic epithelial neoplasms could be designated as thymomas, it has been customary to restrict this term to those neoplasms showing no overt atypia of the epithelial component, and to classify the others as thymic carcinomas (see Sect. 1.2)

The classification of thymomas (by themselves and in relation to thymic carcinomas) has been and remains a source of debate. No consensus has been reached on how to best subdivide these tumours and what terms are to be used for these subtypes. However, some general principles and conclusions have emerged from the various classification schemes proposed over the years.

Historically, there have been two separate approaches to the evaluation and subdivision of thymomas. One has been based on the presence and degree of contiguous invasion, and presence of implants, lymph node metastases or distant metastases, and therefore has incorporated the criteria of a staging system. The other approach has been promulgated on the basis of the cytoarchitectural features of the tumor independently from the presence and degree of invasiveness. A definite correlation exists among the two approaches in that some tumour subtypes are more likely to be invasive (and therefore clinically more aggressive) than others. However, it is important to realize that the two evaluations should be made independently, and that the one based on the invasive/metastasising properties of the tumour relates more closely to recurrence and outcome than the one based on cytoarchitectural features, to the point of markedly reducing the independent prognostic value of the latter. It should be acknowledged that this remains a controversial issue and that additional studies will be necessary to settle it.

According to the first scheme, thymomas are divided, irrespective of cytoarchitectural type, into the following categories:

-   Encapsulated: *A thymoma completely surrounded by a fibrous capsule of varying thickness which is not infiltrated by tumour growth.*

Thymic tumors that infiltrate into, but not through, the capsule still belong in this category.

-   Minimally invasive: *A thymoma surrounded by a capsule which is focally infiltrated by tumour growth or which invades the mediastinal fat.*

The capsular invasion needs to be complete in order for the tumour to be placed in this category. Minimally invasive thymomas are usually identifiable as such only after microscopic examination, insofar as they generally appear to the surgeon indistinguishable from encapsulated thymomas at the time of excision.

-   Widely invasive: *A thymoma spreading by direct extension into adjacent structures such as pericardium, large vessels or lung.*

This type of thymoma usually appears invasive to the surgeon at the time of excision, which may be incomplete as a result.

In addition to the above subdivision, which is dependent upon the presence and degree of *contiguous* tumour spread, the following features of thymoma should be listed in the diagnosis whenever present:

-   With implants: *A thymoma in which tumour nodules separate from the main mass are found on the pericardial or pleural surface.*

These implants tend to be small and multiple and their microscopic appearance is usually, but not always, similar to that of the parent tumour.

-   With lymph node metastases: *A thymoma that involves one or more lymph nodes anatomically separate from the main mass.*

This excludes direct extension into the node by the tumour. The nodes most commonly involved by metastatic thymoma are mediastinal and supraclavicular. It is a rare event even in long-standing cases, but exceptionally it represents the first clinical manifestation of the tumour.

-   With distant metastases: *A thymoma accompanied by embolic metastases to a distant site.*

This excludes metastases to lymph nodes and direct extension into any organ. The sites most commonly involved by embolic metastases are lung, liver and skeletal system.

It may appear peculiar for a "histological " classification to include criteria such as implants or metastases. We feel that this decision is justified because these criteria have a bearing on whether a thymoma is regarded as benign or malignant, in a fashion similar to that used for tumours such as meningioma or paraganglioma. Since these features do not have an equivalent significance in thymic carcinomas (which are malignant by definition), they are listed only for the thymomas, even if their occurrence is obviously of prognostic importance also in thymic carcinomas.

In conventional classification schemes, encapsulated thymomas lacking implants, lymph node metastases, or distant metastases are regarded as *benign*, whereas all other combinations are viewed as *malignant* (sometimes designated as *type I* malignant thymomas to distinguish them from thymic carcinomas, designated in the same scheme as *type II* malignant thymomas). Whereas there is no question that thymomas that are widely invasive and/or that are accompanied by implants, lymph node metastases or distant metastases are to be regarded as malignant on clinical grounds, it is not so apparent that the minimally invasive tumours deserve that appellation, particularly in view of the fact that in multilobated tumours it is often difficult to decide whether "minimal invasion" is present or not.

When evaluating the possibility of thymoma implants being present, it should be remembered that thymomas can develop in ectopic locations outside the anterosuperior mediastinum, including other portions of the mediastinum, pulmonary hilum, pleura and neck.

As already stated, the second approach has been to evaluate these tumours on the combined basis of the morphology of the neoplastic epithelial cells (spindle, plump, etc.) and the relative number of these cells vis-à-vis the non-neoplastic lymphocytic component. Some classifications have used a purely descriptive terminology (e.g. predominantly spindle cell, predominantly lymphocytic, etc.), whereas others have included terms derived from perceived morphologic and "functional" analogies between the various patterns of thymoma and the various compartments of the normal thymus. Since the presence of a bonafide correspondence between a certain thymoma morphology and a given anatomic compartment of the normal thymus (e.g. between a so-called medullary thymoma and normal thymic medulla) has yet to be convincingly demonstrated, the terminology chosen here is a non-committal one based on a combination of letters and numbers. It is not proposed as a new classification, but mainly to facilitate comparison among the many terms and classification schemes that have been offered over the years. It may not be as intuitive as any of those previous schemes, but it will avoid the introduction or perpetuation of possibly inaccurate or at least unproven notions. It is based on the following major criteria:

1. There are two major types of thymoma depending on whether the neoplastic epithelial cells and their nuclei have a spindle/oval shape (here designated as *type A*), or whether these cells have a dendritic or plump ("epithelioid") appearance (here designated as *type B*). Tumours combining these two morphologies are designated as *type AB*.
2. Type B thymomas are further subdivided on the basis of the proportional increase (in relation to the lymphocytes) and emergence of atypia of the neoplastic epithelial cells into three subtypes, respectively designated as *B1*, *B2* and *B3*.

Thymic carcinomas remain named as such, although when viewed within the spectrum of thymic epithelial tumours (to which they certainly belong), they could be regarded as representing type C thymomas. Not unexpectedly, combinations of the above categories can occur within the same tumour. For those cases, a term such as *combined thymoma* can be used, followed by a listing of the various components and their relative amount. The reader may associate the various letters proposed here with the various tumour patterns by mnemonically assuming that "A" stands for atrophic (i.e. the effete thymic cell of adult life), "B" for bioactive (i.e. the biologically active organ of the fetus and infant) and "C" for carcinoma.

As a closing for this introductory section, the Committee wishes to stress again the importance of independently evaluating thymic epithelial tumours on the basis of their presence and degree of invasiveness (using staging criteria) and their cytoarchitectural features, and of using this combined approach to predict behaviour.

Histological Classification
of Tumours of the Thymus

---

[1] Morphology code of the International Classification of Diseases for Oncology
   (ICD-O) and the Systematized Nomenclature of Medicine (SNOMED).
   Behaviour is coded /0 for benign tumours, /3 for malignant tumours, and /1 for
   unspecified, borderline or uncertain behaviour. Tumours in the thymoma group
   may be benign or malignant, depending on whether they are encapsulated or
   invasive; when this is unspecified, they are coded /1.

[2] The italicized numbers are provisional codes proposed for the third edition of
   ICD-O. They should, for the most part, be incorporated into the next edition of
   ICD-O, but they are subject to change.

2   Neuroendocrine Tumours

2.1	*Carcinoid tumour (well-differentiated*	
	neuroendocrine carcinoma)	8240/3
2.1.1	Classic	8240/3
2.1.2	Spindle cell	
2.1.3	Pigmented	
2.1.4	With amyloid (extrathyroidal medullary carcinoma)8511/3	
2.1.5	Atypical	8249/3
2.2	*Small cell carcinoma (poorly differentiated*	
	neuroendocrine carcinoma)	8041/3
2.2.1	Mixed small cell-epidermoid	
	keratinizing carcinoma	*8045/3*
2.3	*Large cell neuroendocrine carcinoma*	*8013/3*

3   Germ Cell Tumours

3.1	*Seminoma (germinoma)*	9061/3
3.2	*Embryonal carcinoma*	9070/3
3.3	*Yolk sac tumour*	9071/3
3.4	*Choriocarcinoma*	9100/3
3.5	*Teratoma*	
3.5.1	Mature teratoma	9080/0
3.5.2	Immature teratoma	9080/3
3.5.3	With sarcoma	9084/3
3.6	*Mixed germ cell tumour*	9085/3

4   Lymphoid Tumours

4.1	*Hodgkin lymphoma*	9650/3
4.1.1	Nodular sclerosis	9663/3
4.2	*Large cell lymphoma*	9680/3
4.2.1	With sclerosis	

Definitions and Explanatory Notes

1 Epithelial Tumours

1.1 Thymoma

1.1.1 Type A thymoma (spindle cell; medullary) (Figs. 1–4)

A tumour composed of a population of neoplastic thymic epithelial cells having spindle/oval shape, lacking nuclear atypia, and accompanied by few or no non-neoplastic lymphocytes.

The appearance of this tumour can simulate that of a mesenchymal neoplasm, but the immunohistochemical and ultrastructural features are clearly those of an epithelial tissue. Rosette-like formations (without a central lumen), foci with a storiform pattern of growth and gland-like formations may be present, the latter often located within or immediately beneath the tumour capsule. The tumour cell nuclei have dispersed to coarse chromatin and inconspicuous nuclei.

Most type A thymomas are encapsulated, but some may invade the capsule, and a few have been seen extending into the lung.

Type A thymomas have been traditionally designated spindle cell thymomas, but not all of the tumour cells have a spindle shape; some are oval and, on occasion, these constitute the bulk of this tumour, while still maintaining the architectural features listed above. Type A thymoma has also been designated *medullary thymoma*, since its cells resemble spindle- and oval-shaped normal thymic medullary epithelial cells at the ultrastructural level, and also because these tumours contain few, if any, immature T lymphocytes. However, one rarely, if ever, finds in this tumour an attempt at Hassall corpuscle formations. Actually, many of the features are more reminiscent of the cells seen in the atrophic thymus of adult life, some of which happen to be located in the subcapsular region.

There are exceptionally rare thymomas composed of spindle cells but exhibiting nuclear hyperchromasia, pleomorphism, mitotic activity and/or necrosis. It is not clear whether they should be regarded as atypical or poorly differentiated forms of type A thymomas, as "spindle cell variants" of type B3 thymomas, or as sarcomatoid (spindle cell) thymic carcinomas. Clues to their recognition include a prominent reticulin fibre network among individual tumour cells and a lack or paucity of palisading cells around perivascular spaces.

1.1.2   Type AB thymoma (mixed) (Figs. 5–7)

A tumour in which foci having the features of type A thymoma are admixed with foci rich in lymphocytes.

The segregation of the two patterns can be sharp or indistinct, and there is a wide range in the relative amount of the two components. In particular, type A areas can be extremely scant. The neoplastic epithelial cells in the lymphocyte-rich areas tend to be plumper than those in the lymphocyte-poor foci, which can be easily misinterpreted as hypercellular fibrous septa. Any of the features described in type A thymomas can be found in the homologous areas of the type AB tumours. Similarly, features usually absent in type A thymomas (such as Hassall corpuscles) are also lacking in the type A component of these tumours.

The term "mixed" often applied to this tumour is meant by some to simply indicate a mixed population of epithelial cells and lymphocytes, and by others (in a more restricted and precise way) to highlight the admixture of foci resembling normal thymic medulla (the lymphocyte-poor areas) and normal thymic cortex (the lymphocyte-rich areas). The objections raised to the latter assumption in connection to type A thymomas also apply here.

1.1.3   Type B1 thymoma (lymphocyte-rich; lymphocytic; predominantly cortical; organoid) (Figs. 8–13)

A tumour which resembles the normal functional thymus in that it combines large expanses having an appearance practically indistinguishable from normal thymic cortex with areas resembling thymic medulla.

The resemblance between this tumour type and the normal active thymus is such that the distinction between the two may be impossible on high-power examination. This also applies to the neoplastic epithelial cells, the nuclei of which are vesicular, with distinct small nucleoli. The areas of "medullary differentiation" appear as lighter round foci that can simulate germinal centres. Occasionally, these are seen to contain a cluster of squamoid epithelial cells in their centre, or fully developed Hassall corpuscles. Perivascular spaces may be present, although as a rule they are not as numerous or well-developed as those seen in types B2 or B3 thymomas. In contrast to the situation with other thymoma types, most of the various terms that have been applied over the years to type B1 thymomas are reasonably accurate: They certainly are *lymphocyte-rich*, they display striking *organoid* features in that they closely resemble the normal organ, and they are *predominantly cortical*, in that there is a predominance of areas resembling cortex over those resembling medulla. A less accurate term is *lymphocytic thymoma*, in that it implies a lymphocytic derivation for a tumour which – like all other thymomas – is of epithelial nature. Indeed, close inspection at high power will often reveal subtle abnormalities in the size and distribution of the epithelial cells, which – when more pronounced – result in a merging with those seen in type B2 tumours.

1.1.4   *Type B2 thymoma (cortical)* (Figs. 14–16)

A tumour in which the neoplastic epithelial component appears as scattered plump cells with vesicular nuclei and distinct nucleoli among a heavy population of lymphocytes. Perivascular spaces are common and sometimes very prominent. A perivascular arrangement of tumour cells resulting in a palisading effect may be seen.

Type B2 thymoma resembles type B1 thymoma in its predominance of lymphocytes, but foci of medullary differentiation are less conspicuous or absent. Hassall corpuscles may be seen within these medullary foci, and therefore their presence does not necessarily place a thymoma into the type B1 category.

The epithelial cells of type B2 thymomas are more numerous than in the type B1 tumour and have a more obvious neoplastic appearance by virtue of their enlarged vesicular nuclei and conspicuous nucleoli. The cytoplasm tends to be abundant and the shape of the cells round or polygonal, this feature having led to the alternative designation *(large) polygonal cell thymoma*. Sometimes, these cells arrange themselves in tight clusters. Some or most of the lymphocytes may have an immature appearance, manifested by enlarged nuclear size, open chromatin pattern, visible cytoplasm and mitotic activity.

Like B1 thymoma, type B2 thymoma is lymphocyte-rich, albeit to a lesser degree, this resulting in a mixed lymphocyte-epithelial pattern in some cases. This tumour is sometimes designated as cortical, but in reality it is not more so than the type B1 tumour. Its differences with the former rather depend on the fact that it is a lesser differentiated tumour, no longer able to recapitulate the cortico-medullary compartments of the normal thymus to the extent that the B1 thymoma does, and exhibiting a morphologically and/or numerically distinctly abnormal population of epithelial cells.

1.1.5   Type B3 thymoma (epithelial; atypical; squamoid; well-differentiated thymic carcinoma) (Figs. 17–22)

A type of thymoma predominantly composed of epithelial cells having a round or polygonal shape and exhibiting no or mild atypia. They are admixed with a minor component of lymphocytes, resulting in a sheet-like growth of the neoplastic epithelial cells.

Type B3 thymoma shares with type A thymoma a predominantly or almost exclusively epithelial composition, but differs from it in the fact that the shape of the cell is round or polygonal rather than spindle or oval. These cells may be either small and polygonal, with small round nuclei and inconspicuous nucleoli, or large, with nuclei and nucleoli resembling those of type B2 thymomas. Any of the architectural features seen in the latter (such as perivascular spaces and perivascular arrangement of tumour cells) can also be encountered in B3 thymomas. Squamoid or squamous foci are more common than in the latter.

This thymoma type has been traditionally known as *epithelial*, a term which is accurate but somewhat misleading since it implies that the other types of thymoma are not. Another term that has been suggested for it is *atypical*, but this is also somewhat inaccurate in view of the fact that the degree of atypia present in it may not be greater than that seen in type B2 thymoma, from which it is distinguished primarily on the basis of the proportionally larger number of epithelial cells. A further proposal is that of *well-differentiated thymic carcinoma*, which is potentially confusing because of the fact that in most articles on the subject and in most classification schemes this tumour is included with the thymomas rather than with the thymic carcinomas. Yet another proposal is that of *squamoid thymoma* because of the common presence of squamoid or squamous features in the tumour cells. However, this is neither a constant nor an exclusive feature of this tumour type.

1.2   Thymic carcinoma (type C thymoma)

A thymic tumour exhibiting clear-cut cytologic atypia and a set of cytoarchitectural features no longer specific to the thymus (as for types A, AB and B thymomas), but rather analogous to those seen in carcinomas of other organs. In contrast to thymomas in the A and/or B categories, type C thymomas (thymic carcinomas) lack immature lymphocytes; whatever lymphocytes may be present are mature and usually admixed with plasma cells.

1.2.1   Epidermoid keratinizing (squamous cell) carcinoma
(Figs. 23–25)

A type of thymic carcinoma exhibiting clear-cut cytologic atypia and equally clear-cut evidence of squamous differentiation in routinely stained sections, in the form of intercellular bridges and/or squamous pearls.

An architectural feature which constitutes an important diagnostic clue in the differential diagnosis with squamous cell carcinomas of other sites is the common presence of prominent interconnected lobules separated by sharply delineated fibrohyaline bands infiltrated by inflammatory cells. Theoretically, these tumours could be graded microscopically following criteria analogous to those employed for squamous cell carcinomas in other sites, such as upper or lower respiratory tract.

1.2.2   Epidermoid non-keratinizing carcinoma (Figs. 26–28)

A type of thymic carcinoma composed of large epithelial cells exhibiting clear-cut cytologic atypia but lacking overt signs of keratinization in routinely stained sections.

The overall appearance is similar to that of tumours in the previous category, but the lobulation is less developed or altogether absent.

Epidermoid thymic carcinomas (whether keratinizing or non-keratinizing are immunoreactive for CD5 in nearly all cases and for the neuroendocrine markers chromogranin and synaptophysin in about half of the cases, whereas thymomas are usually negative for all three markers

1.2.3   Lymphoepithelioma-like carcinoma (Fig. 29)

A type of thymic carcinoma having morphologic features indistinguishable from those of lymphoepithelial carcinoma of the upper respiratory tract (see WHO Histological Typing of Tumours of the Upper Respiratory Tract and Ear).

This tumour has a characteristic syncytial pattern of growth. The tumour cells have large nuclei with very prominent, sharply outlined nucleoli. There is a heavy inflammatory infiltrate, of predominantly lymphocytic nature, which may freely intermingle with the tumour cells or be grouped in small clusters. This tumour needs to be distinguished from germ cell tumours of both seminoma and embryonal carcinoma types.

1.2.4   Sarcomatoid carcinoma (carcinosarcoma) (Figs. 30–32)

A type of thymic carcinoma in which part or all of the tumour resembles one of the types of soft tissue sarcoma.

The tumour may be entirely composed of sarcoma-like areas, or these may be admixed with foci having a carcinomatous appearance (so-called carcinosarcoma). The tumour cells may be spindle-shaped or highly pleomorphic. Specific lines of mesenchymal differentiation may be encountered, such as skeletal muscle fibres or cartilage.

1.2.5   Clear cell carcinoma (Fig. 33)

A type of thymic carcinoma composed predominantly or exclusively of cells with optically clear cytoplasm.

The pattern of growth is generally solid and there is often marked nuclear atypia. The main differential diagnosis is with metastatic renal cell carcinoma.

1.2.6   Basaloid carcinoma (Fig. 34)

A type of thymic carcinoma composed of compact lobules of tumour cells exhibiting peripheral palisading and an overall basophilic staining pattern due to the high nucleo-cytoplasmic ratio and the absence of keratinization.

This tumour often presents as a mural nodule in a thymic cyst.

1.2.7   Mucoepidermoid carcinoma (Fig. 35)

A type of thymic carcinoma having an appearance similar to that of mucoepidermoid carcinoma of major or minor salivary glands.

Both the squamous and the mucin-producing components should be cytologically well-differentiated for a tumour to be placed into this category. A component of "intermediate" cells is also usually present.

In agreement with the policy followed in other organs (such as lung), carcinomas containing poorly differentiated squamous and glandular elements should be called *adenosquamous carcinomas* rather than mucoepidermoid carcinomas. Such tumours probably exist in the thymus, but have not yet been properly characterised.

1.2.8   Papillary carcinoma (Fig. 36)

A type of thymic carcinoma growing in a papillary fashion. This may be accompanied by psammoma body formation, resulting in a marked similarity with papillary carcinoma of the thyroid gland.

Some of the examples of this exceptionally rare type of thymic carcinoma have been seen admixed with type A thymoma, suggesting an origin from the latter.

1.2.9   Undifferentiated carcinoma

A type of thymic carcinoma growing in a solid undifferentiated fashion but without exhibiting sarcomatoid (spindle cell or pleomorphic) features.

The diagnosis of this exceptionally rare type of thymic carcinoma is always one of exclusion, and it usually requires confirmation of its epithelial nature through immunohistochemical and/or ultrastructural evaluation.

2   Neuroendocrine Tumours

Thymic tumours should be placed into this category only when the neuroendocrine elements constitute the predominant or exclusive component of the neoplasm. This category should not be used for otherwise typical thymic carcinomas (type C thymomas) containing neuroendocrine cells, a feature present in over half of the cases.

2.1   Carcinoid tumour
(well-differentiated neuroendocrine carcinoma)

A well-differentiated tumour composed of a uniform population of cells growing in the form of neuroendocrine-type nests, glands, ribbons and festoons, and in which neuroendocrine differentiation can be demonstrated immunohistochemically or ultrastructurally.

In general, the neuroendocrine differentiation in these tumours can be easily demonstrated with pan-neuroendocrine markers (such as chromogranin or synaptophysin) or through the ultrastructural identification of neurosecretory granules. Mitotic activity is low and necrosis is scanty or absent.

2.1.1   *Classic carcinoid* (Figs. 37, 38)

A carcinoid tumour comprised of polygonal cells with granular amphophilic cytoplasm. Ribbons, festoons, solid nests and rosette-like glands are common.

Despite the well-differentiated nature of the tumour, stromal and vascular invasion are often present. High vascularity is a constant feature. Mitoses and necrosis are practically absent.

2.1.2   *Spindle cell carcinoid* (Fig. 39)

A carcinoid tumour comprised of spindle cells, often arranged in fascicles.

This tumour type is morphologically identical to the homonymous tumour of lung. Occasionally, it is found admixed with a carcinoid tumour of the classic type.

2.1.3   *Pigmented carcinoid* (Fig. 40)

A carcinoid tumour in which some of the tumour cells contain intracytoplasmic melanin.

Some of the melanin granules are found within the cytoplasm of histiocytes, and these have a coarser quality.

2.1.4   With amyloid (extrathyroidal medullary carcinoma) (Fig. 41)

A well-differentiated neuroendocrine carcinoma accompanied by amyloid deposition in the stroma.

The tumour cells are usually spindle-shaped and immunoreactive for calcitonin. Thus, the tumour is indistinguishable from medullary carcinoma of the thyroid gland and probably composed of extra-thyroidal C cells.

2.1.5   Atypical carcinoid (Fig. 42)

A carcinoid tumour retaining the architectural features of the classic type but exhibiting a greater degree of mitotic activity and/or foci of necrosis, which tend to appear as sharply outlined ("punctate") areas in the centre of the tumor nests.

The criteria for the identification of this tumour are the same as for the homonymous lung neoplasm. This includes a mitotic count of 2–10/2 mm^2 (10 hpf). The proportion of thymic carcinoid tumours falling into the "atypical" category is higher than for pulmonary carcinoid tumours.

2.2   Small cell carcinoma (poorly differentiated neuroendocrine carcinoma) (Fig. 43)

A high-grade thymic tumour having morphologic features indistinguishable from those of the homonymous lung tumour. Evidence of neuroendocrine differentiation is usually found on ultrastructural or immunohistochemical examination.

The alternative possibility of a mediastinal metastasis from a primary pulmonary neoplasm should always be considered before making a diagnosis of primary small cell carcinoma of thymus.

2.2.1   Mixed small cell-epidermoid keratinizing carcinoma (Fig. 44)

A high-grade malignant thymic tumour combining features of small cell carcinoma and epidermoid keratinizing thymic carcinoma.

The two components of this tumour tend to be sharply segregated. The appearance is similar to that seen in the homonymous lung neoplasm.

2.3   Large cell neuroendocrine carcinoma

A high-grade malignant thymic tumour composed of large cells exhibiting neuroendocrine features and containing a large number of mitotic figures. Necrosis is present, often in the form of extensive foci.

The main differential feature between this tumour and "atypical carcinoid" (see Sect. 2.1.5) is the mitotic count, as is also the case for their pulmonary counterparts. Neuroendocrine-type architectural features are likely to be not as prominently displayed as in the better differentiated forms of neuroendocrine carcinoma.

3   Germ Cell Tumours (Figs. 45, 46)

The terminology recommended for these tumours is the same as for germ cell tumours of testis and ovary (see corresponding WHO classifications). The large majority of primary mediastinal germ cell tumours arise within or in close proximity to the thymus, but mediastinal mature teratomas have also been reported in an intrapericardial location. *Seminomas (germinomas)* of the thymus are for all practical purposes restricted to males. Like seminomas of testis, they are associated with inflammation and sometimes a brisk granulomatous response. They can also elicit prominent cystic transformation of the thymic epithelium, a condition known as multilocular thymic cyst (see Sect. 6.3).

Germ cell tumours of the thymus can be accompanied by a sarcomatous component (such as *angiosarcoma* or *rhabdomyosarcoma*), a complication of grave prognostic significance since this neoplastic component is not likely to respond to germ cell tumour-type chemotherapeutic protocols.

4   Lymphoid Tumours (Figs. 47–55)

The nomenclature to be used for these tumours when involving the thymus is the same as that recommended in the WHO classification on the subject.

In this publication, the only lymphoma types listed are those known to affect the thymus as the only or predominant site, in order of frequency. The three most common types are Hodgkin lymphoma, large cell lymphoma and lymphoblastic lymphoma. *Hodgkin lymphoma* is nearly always of nodular sclerosis type and is often accompanied by cystic transformation of the thymic epithelium (so-called multilocular thymic cyst; see Sect. 6.3). In the past, cases of Hodgkin lymphoma of the thymus were mistakenly regarded by some as of thymic epithelial origin and designated as granulomatous thymomas. Exceptional instances of coexistent true thymoma and Hodgkin lymphoma of the thymus have been described.

Large cell lymphoma is characteristically of B-cell type. It is often accompanied by prominent fibrosis ("large cell lymphoma with sclerosis"), which may lead to a nesting pattern simulating seminoma and other non-lymphoid tumours.

Lymphoblastic lymphoma is a tumour of T or null lymphocytes comprised of small cells with characteristic nuclear convolutions.

Mucosa-associated lymphoid tissue (MALT)-type lymphoma is a low-grade lymphoma of small B lymphocytes, analogous to that seen more often in the gastrointestinal tract or lung.

5   Stromal Tumours

5.1   Thymolipoma (Fig. 56)

A well-circumscribed thymic mass composed of mature adipose tissue and islands of microscopically unremarkable thymic parenchyma.

It is not clear whether thymolipoma is a neoplasm, as opposed to a true thymic hyperplasia that has undergone fatty involution.

5.2   Thymoliposarcoma (Fig. 57)

A malignant tumour having the features of liposarcoma entrapping lobules of thymic parenchyma and exhibiting an intimate anatomic relationship with the thymic stroma.

The liposarcoma is of the well-differentiated type, with the pleomorphic tumour cells having a tendency to align beneath the thymic lobules.

5.3   Solitary fibrous tumour (Fig. 58)

A mesenchymal tumour composed of spindle cells of fibroblastic appearance featuring an admixture of hyper- and hypocellular foci, separated by dense collagen.

This tumour, formerly known as solitary fibrous mesothelioma, can occur anywhere in the mediastinum. It should be regarded as of probable thymic origin only when centered in the thymus and entrapping thymic parenchyma. Benign and malignant forms exist, the latter characterised by high mitotic activity and necrosis.

5.4   Rhabdoid tumour (Fig. 59)

A malignant neoplasm composed of oval to round small cells with their cytoplasm occupied by a homogeneous acidophilic ("hyaline") material which displaces the nucleus to the periphery of the cell.

The "hyaline" appearance of the cytoplasm is due to the accumulation of intermediate filaments composed of vimentin and/or keratin. It seems likely that the rhabdoid appearance is a phenotype which can be exhibited by a variety of tumour cell types rather than a specific entity.

6   Tumour-like Lesions

6.1   True thymic hyperplasia (Fig. 60)

An abnormality of the thymus in which the organ is microscopically unremarkable, but whose weight and/or volume exceed the upper limits of normal for that particular age group.

It is believed that most cases of this ill-defined condition are acquired, rather than representing a failure of involution.

6.2   Lymphoid hyperplasia (lymphofollicular thymitis) (Fig. 61)

An abnormality of the thymus in which secondary lymphoid follicles with germinal centres are easily found in an otherwise normal organ.

The size of the organ may be within normal limits or increased. Isolated lymphoid follicles are a normal occurrence in the infantile thymus, and therefore the diagnosis of lymphoid hyperplasia should be made only when these follicles are found later in life and in relative abundance.

6.3   Multilocular thymic cyst (Figs. 50, 62, 63)

A multicystic transformation of the thymic epithelium, usually accompanied by secondary lymphoid follicles and prominent secondary degenerative changes.

This is an acquired disorder probably induced by the presence of an inflammatory lymphoid infiltrate. The etiology usually remains undetermined, but some cases have been reported secondary to HIV infection. Multilocular thymic cyst can also occur in conjunction with thymic tumours (notably nodular sclerosis Hodgkin lymphoma and seminoma), presumably as a result of the inflammatory component that regularly accompanies them.

6.4   Langerhans cell histiocytosis (Fig. 64)

A proliferative process primarily composed of Langerhans cells, with a variable but sometimes secondary component of eosinophils and macrophages.

The thymus may be involved as the sole manifestation of the disease or as a part of a multisystem process. Controversy still exists as to whether this process should be regarded as reactive or neoplastic. The fact that the Langerhans cell population has been found to be clonal has been used as an argument in favour of the latter.

7   Neck Tumours of Thymic or Related Branchial Pouch Derivation

7.1   Ectopic hamartomatous thymoma (Fig. 65)

A benign tumour of the neck composed of epithelial spindle cells, solid or cystic epithelial islands, and adipose tissue, which intermingle haphazardly to impart a hamartomatous quality.

This tumour characteristically occurs in the supraclavicular region and shows a marked male predilection.

7.2   Ectopic cervical thymoma (Fig. 66)

A tumour having morphologic features analogous to those of thymomas (see Sect. 1.1), but located in the cervical region and not connected with the mediastinal thymus.

Most of these tumours are located within or close to the thyroid. Most reported cases have been type AB (mixed) and non-invasive. There is a marked female predilection

7.3   Spindle epithelial tumour with thymus-like differentiation (SETTLE) (Figs. 67, 68)

A highly cellular tumour of the neck comprised of compact bundles of long spindle epithelial cells which merge with tubulopapillary structures and/or mucinous glands.

Most of these rare tumours have been seen in or around the thyroid gland of children or adolescents. They have a propensity for late distant metastases.

7.4   Carcinoma showing thymus-like differentiation (CASTLE) (Figs. 69, 70)

A malignant tumour of the neck histologically similar to thymic carcinoma and probably representing its ectopic counterpart.

Most reported cases have been of either keratinizing or non-keratinizing type. They have been characterised by a tendency to local recurrence and occasional nodal and distant metastases.

8   Metastatic Tumours

The thymus can be directly involved by primary or secondary tumours involving the mediastinum (particularly lung carcinoma), but is only rarely affected by blood-borne metastases from distant sites.

9   Unclassified Tumours

This group is comprised of tumours which cannot be placed in any of the previously listed categories.

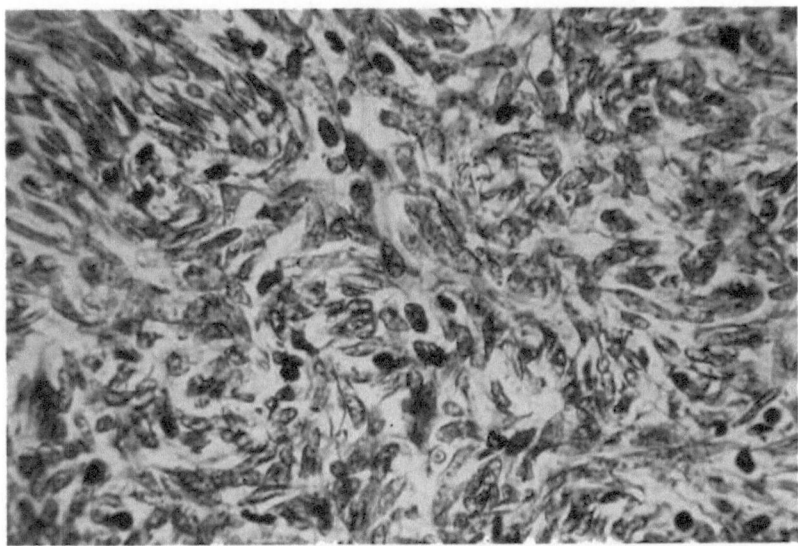

Fig. 1. *Type A thymoma*. Cells with oval-to-spindle nuclei having bland nuclear features. Few lymphocytes

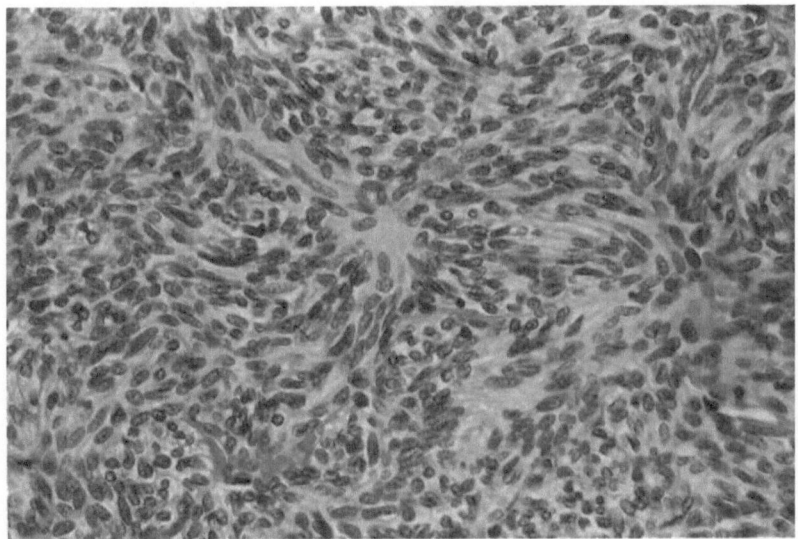

Fig. 2. *Type A thymoma*. Vaguely storiform pattern. Almost complete absence of lymphocytes

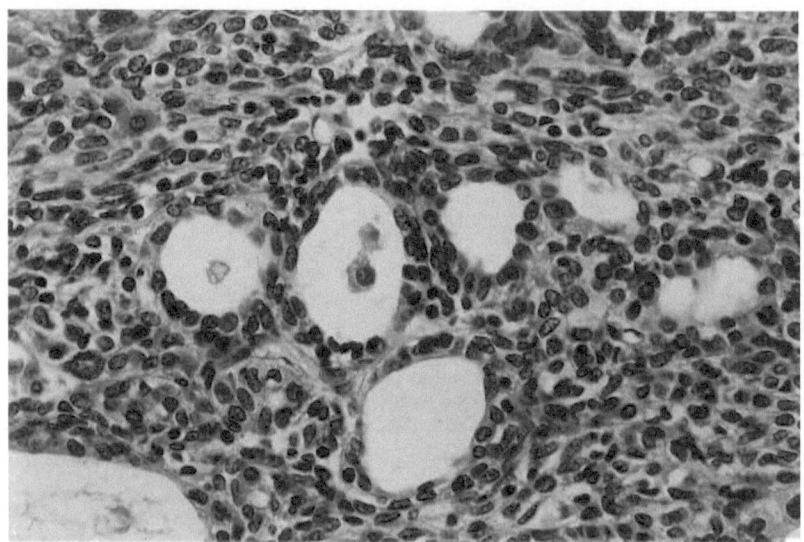

Fig. 3. *Type A thymoma.* Gland-like formations lined by cuboidal cells

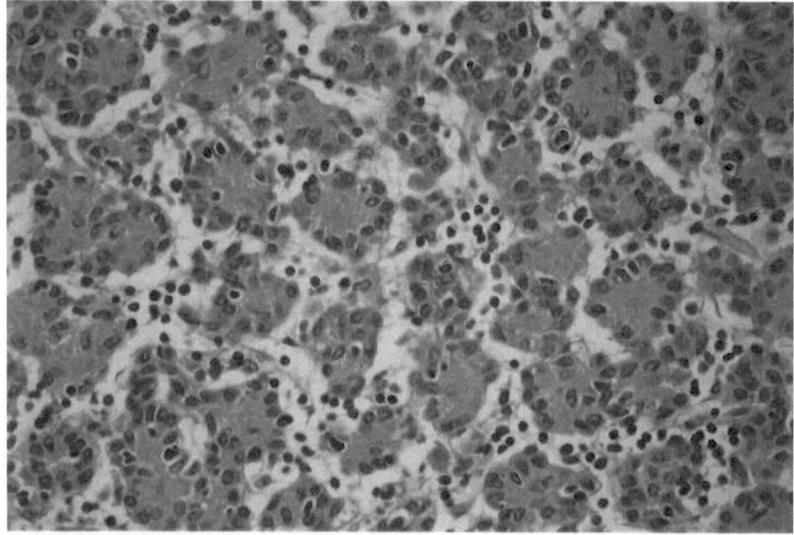

Fig. 4. *Type A thymoma.* Well-defined rosettes without a central lumen. Few lymphocytes in between the tumour cells

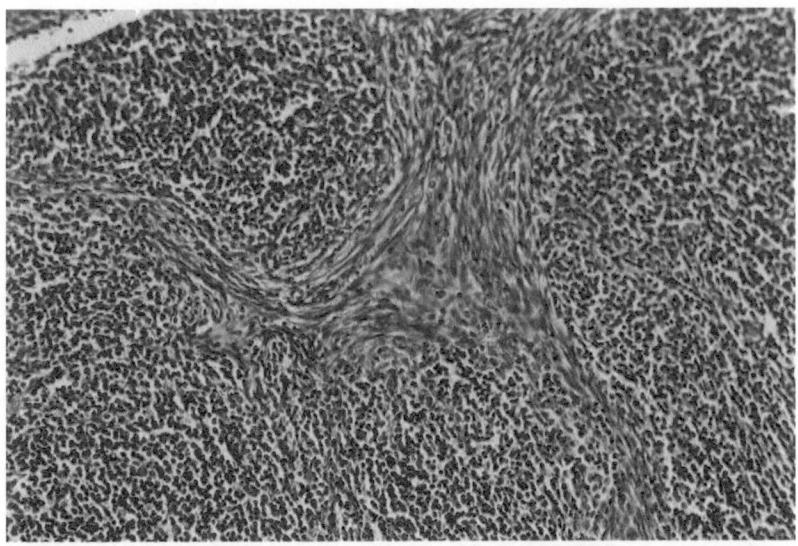

Fig. 5. *Type AB thymoma.* Lymphocyte-rich tumour islands separated by bundles of spindle tumour cells

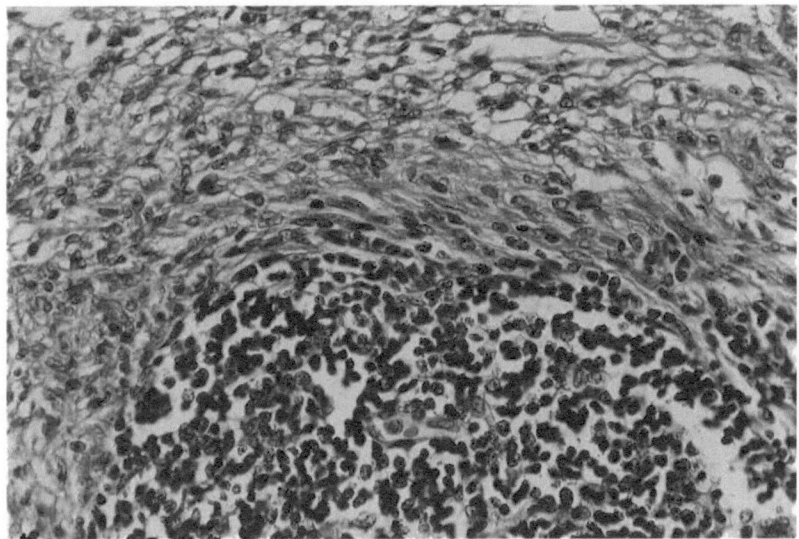

Fig. 6. *Type AB thymoma.* Interface between a lymphocyte-rich area and the lymphocyte-poor spindle cell component similar to that of type A thymoma

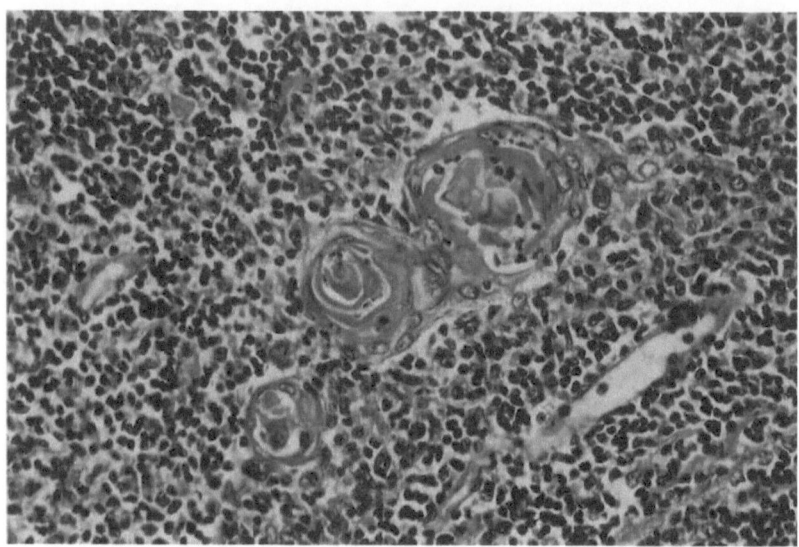

Fig. 7. *Type AB thymoma*. Hassall corpuscle differentiation in the centre of one of the lymphocyte-rich nodules

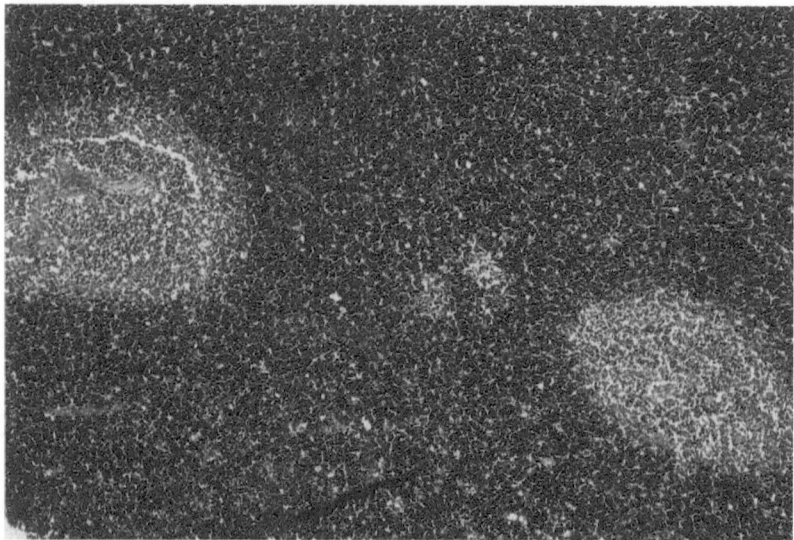

Fig. 8. *Type B1 thymoma*. Marked predominance of lymphocytes. Two areas of medullary differentiation appear as sharply-outlined lighter foci

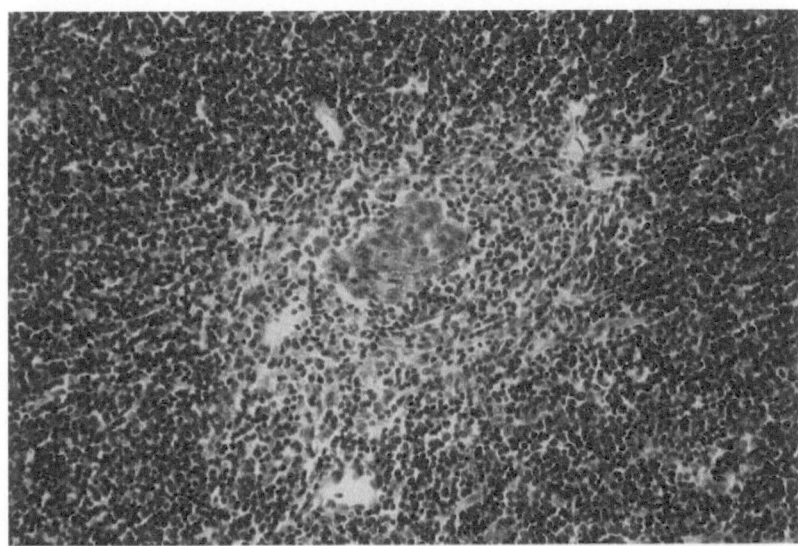

Fig. 9. *Type B1 thymoma.* Area of medullary differentiation showing a cluster of epithelial cells at its very centre, possibly representing an abortive attempt at Hassall corpuscle formation

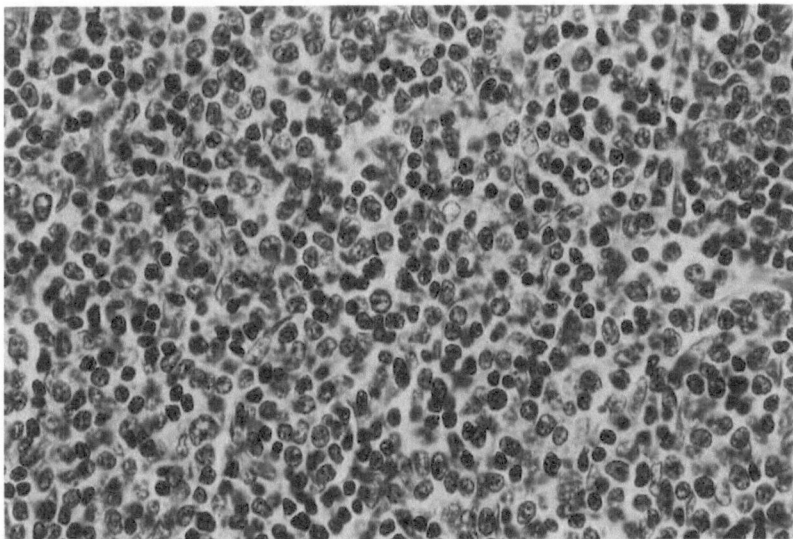

Fig. 10. *Type B1 thymoma.* The predominance of lymphocytes is such as to obscure the thymic epithelial neoplastic component

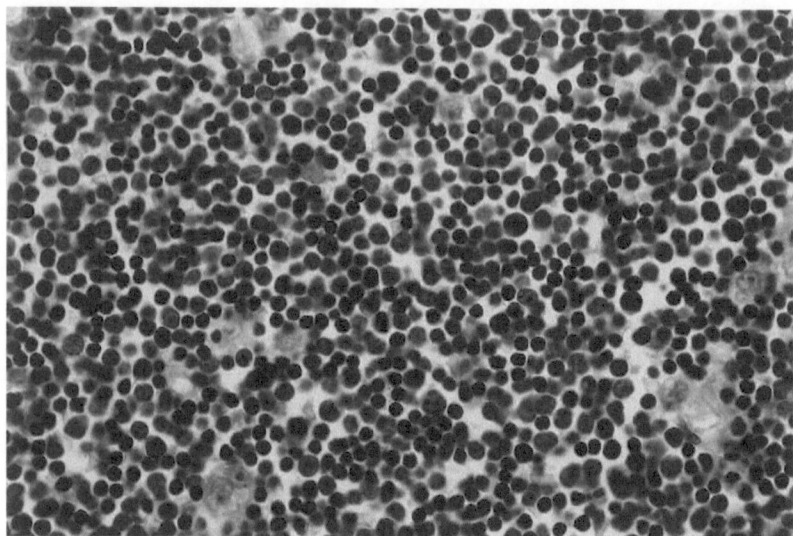

Fig. 11. *Type B1 thymoma.* A few neoplastic epithelial cells are barely visible in a sea of small lymphocytes

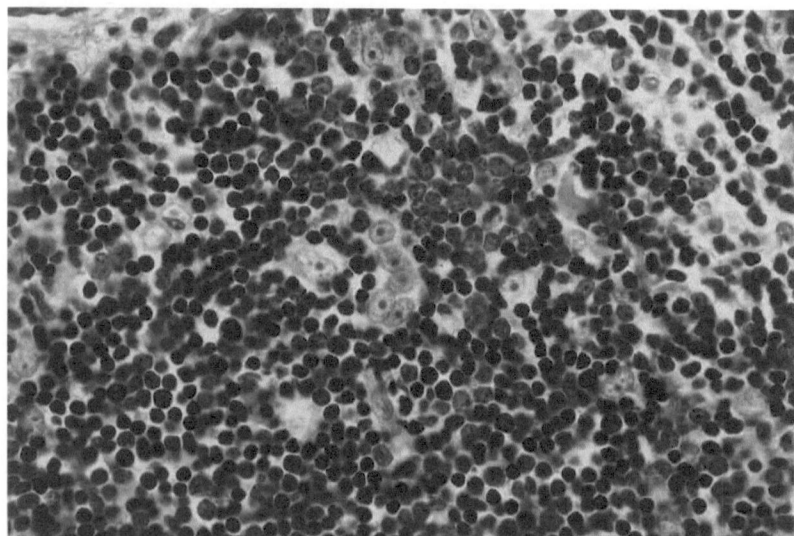

Fig. 12. *Type B1 thymoma.* Another area from the same tumour shown in Fig. 11 is more easily recognisable as a thymoma because of the occasional clustering of the neoplastic epithelial cells

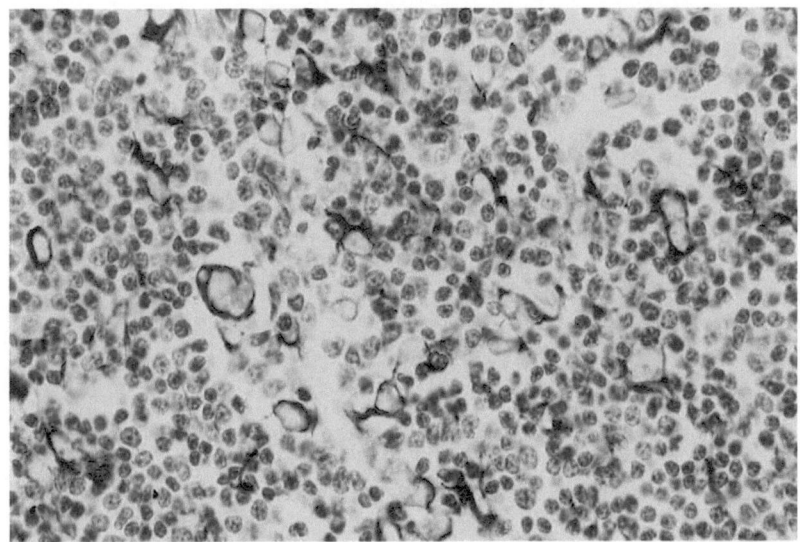

Fig. 13. *Type B1 thymoma.* The keratin stain shows positivity in the cytoplasm and the cytoplasmic prolongations of the tumour cells. This "dendritic" pattern of staining is very characteristic of B1 thymomas

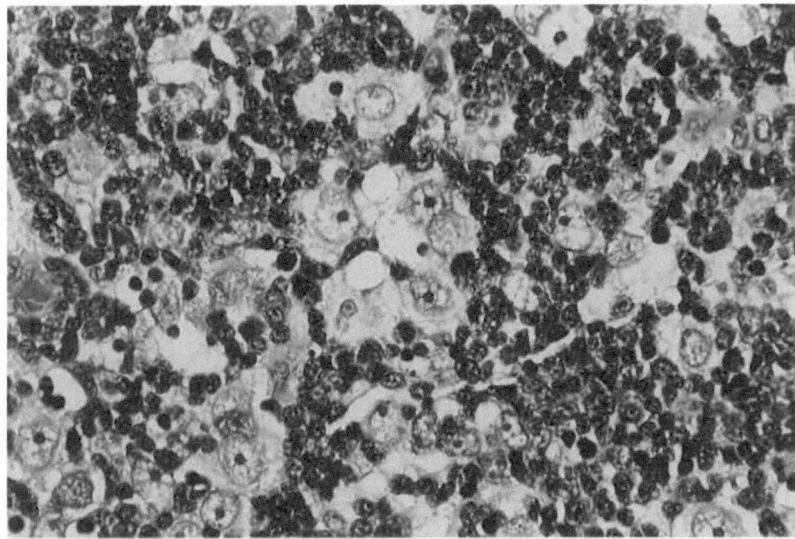

Fig. 14. *Type B2 thymoma.* Predominance of lymphocytes, but epithelial cells are clearly visible and morphologically abnormal by virtue of the nuclear enlargement and nucleolar prominence

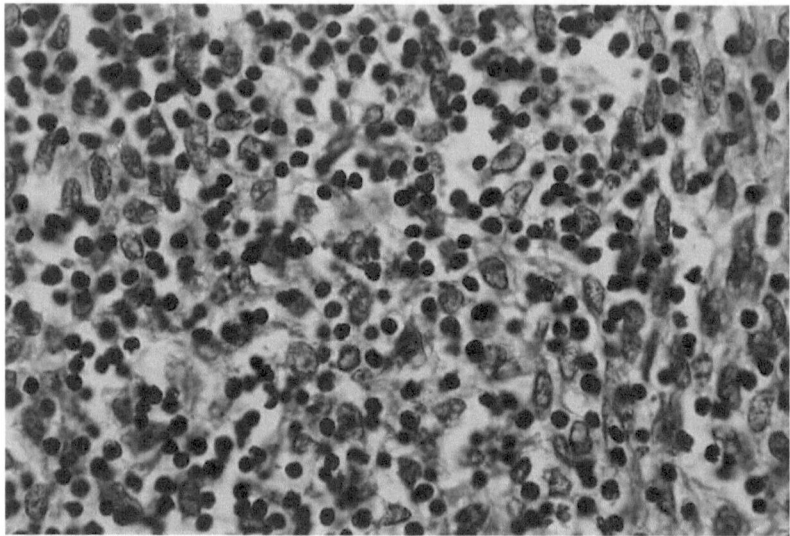

Fig. 15. *Type B2 thymoma.* A relatively even proportion of epithelial cells and lymphocytes, the former exhibiting subtle nuclear abnormalities

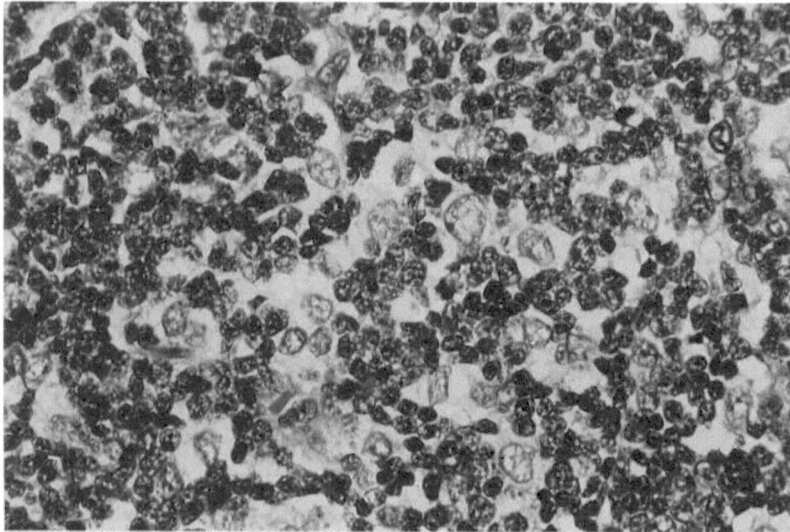

Fig. 16. *Type B2 thymoma.* The neoplastic epithelial cells, which represent a minority of the cell population, show some degree of nuclear pleomorphism

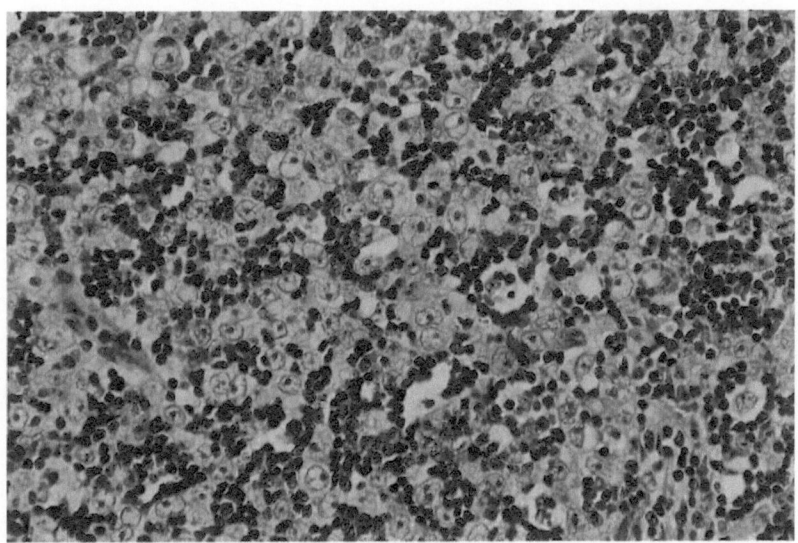

Fig. 17. *Type B3 thymoma.* Predominance of neoplastic epithelial cells, but also a clearly identifiable epithelial lymphocytic component

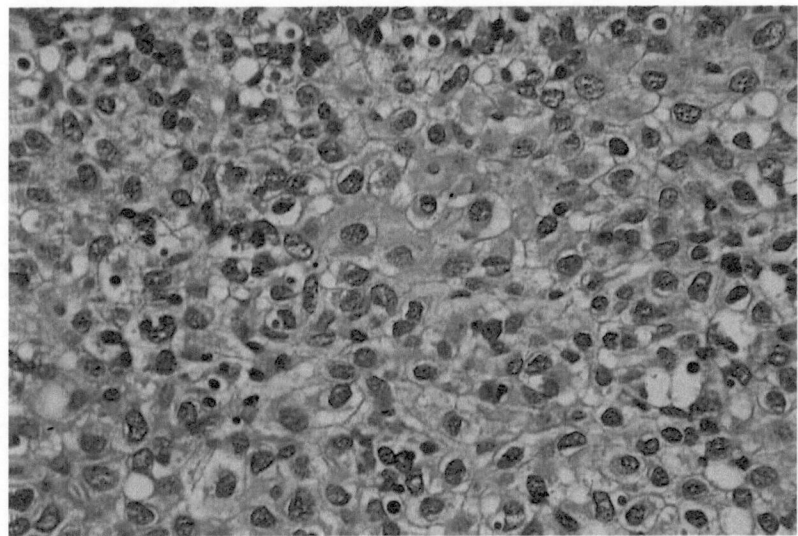

Fig. 18. *Type B3 thymoma.* Solid sheet of tumour cells. Nuclei are rather small and inconspicuous

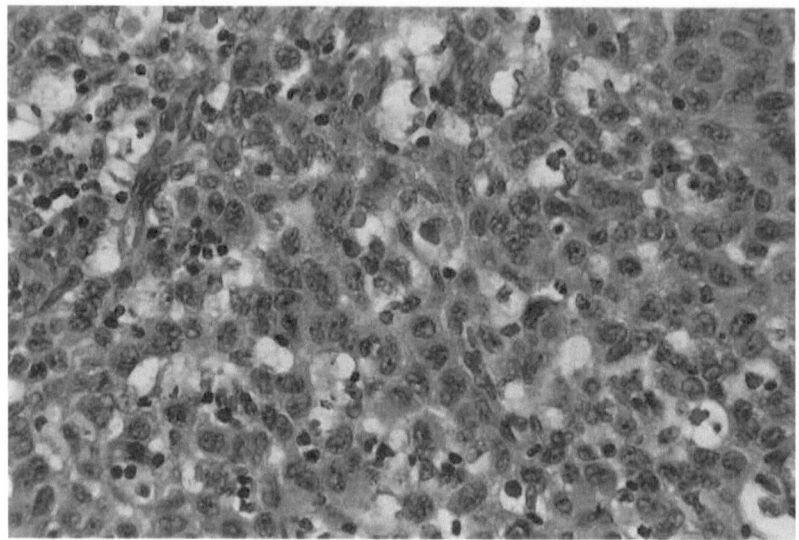

Fig. 19. *Type B3 thymoma.* Great predominance of neoplastic epithelial cells, which show only subtle nuclear aberrations

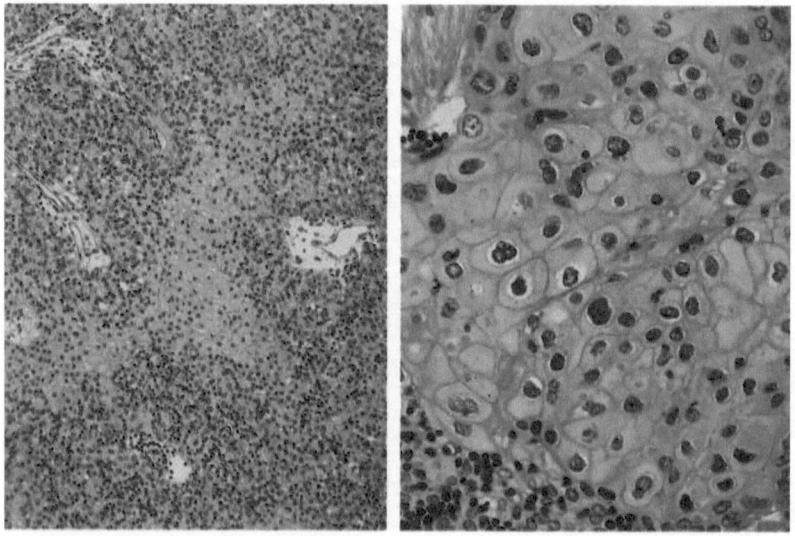

Fig. 20. *Type B3 malignant thymoma.* Some tumour cells show squamoid features, particularly well seen in the high-power view on the right

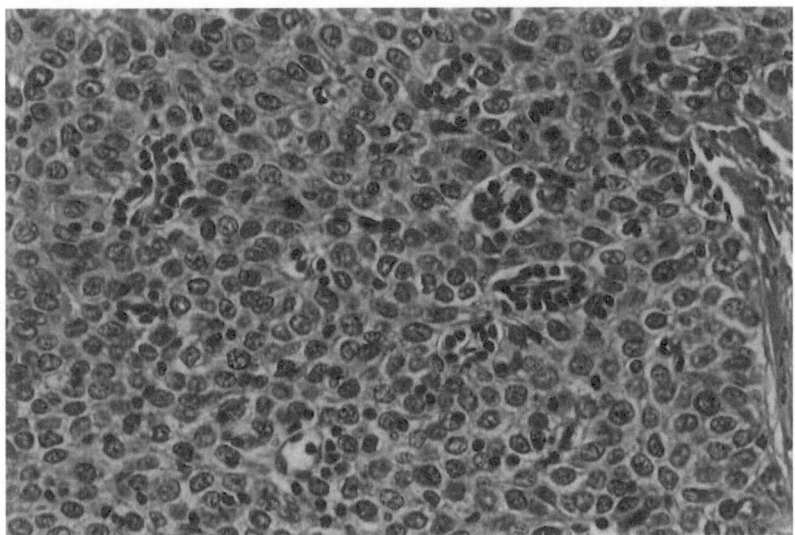

Fig. 21. *Type B3 thymoma.* A solid proliferation of neoplastic epithelial cells is interrupted by a few perivascular collections of lymphocytes

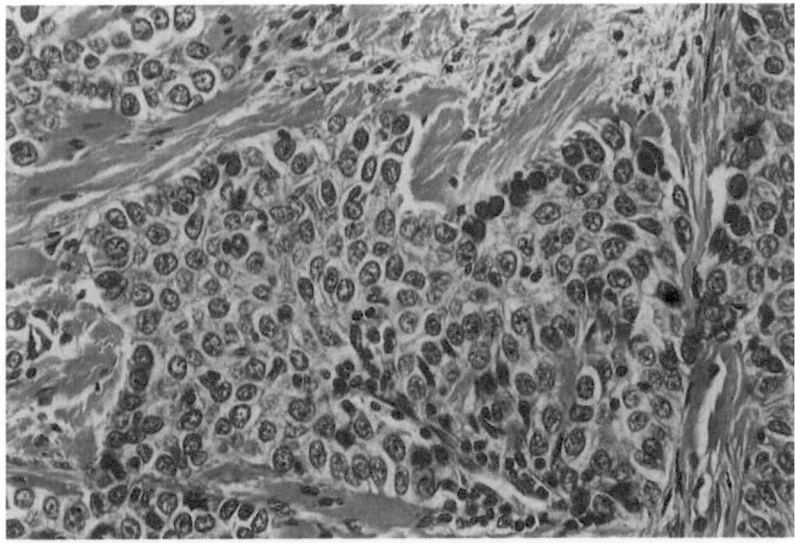

Fig. 22. *Type B3 thymoma.* A sharply outlined cluster of tumour cells accompanied by only a few lymphocytes is bound by hyalinised fibrous bands

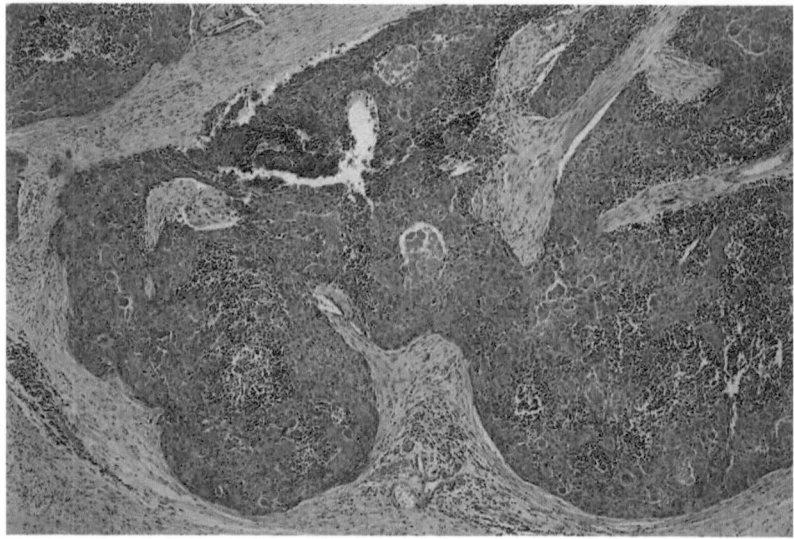

Fig. 23. *Thymic carcinoma, epidermoid keratinizing (squamous cell).* Irregularly-shaped tumour lobules separated by wide fibrous bands

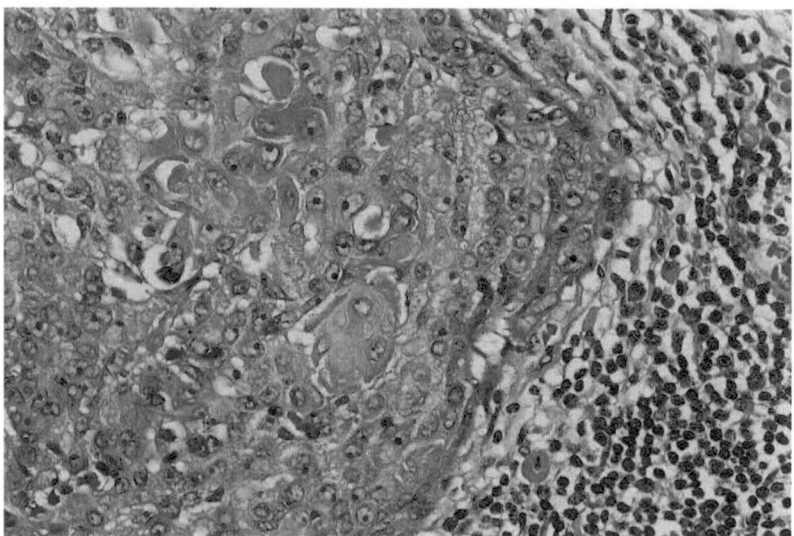

Fig. 24. *Thymic carcinoma, epidermoid keratinizing (squamous cell).* Clear-cut evidence of keratinization towards the centre of the tumour nodule. Fibrous septum on the right infiltrated by lymphocytes

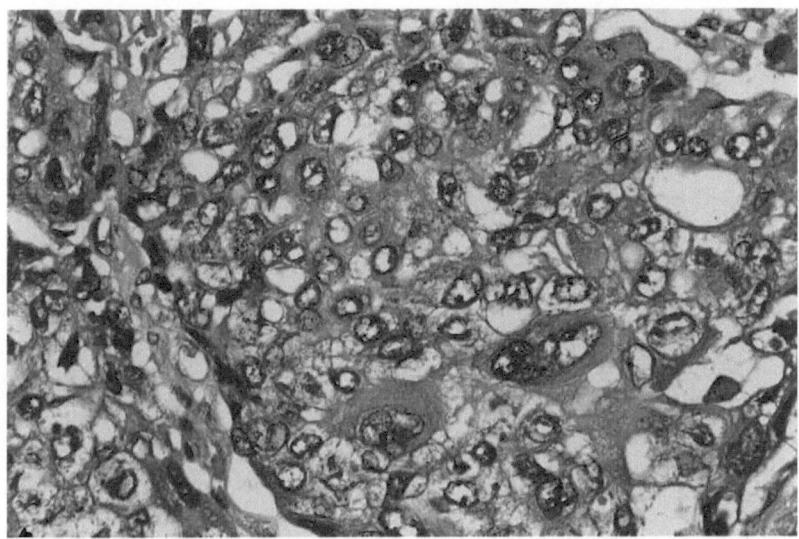

Fig. 25. *Thymic carcinoma, epidermoid keratinizing (squamous cell).* Some keratinizing cells show markedly enlarged hyperchromatic nuclei

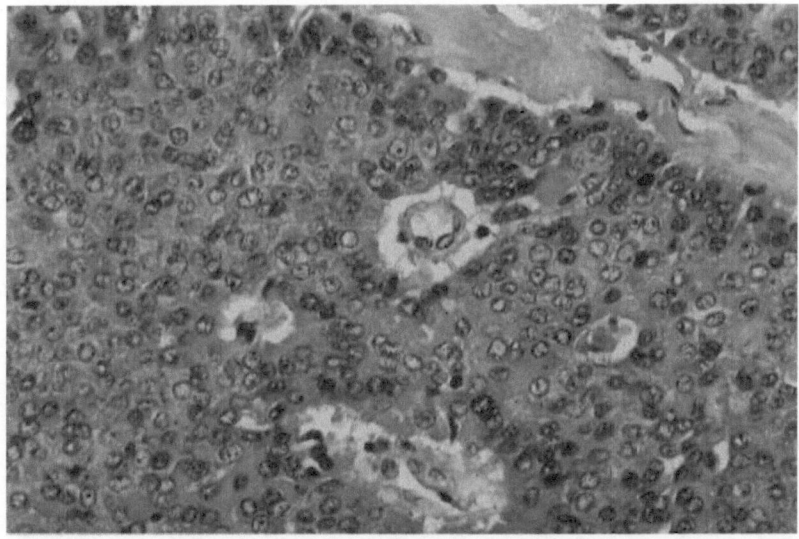

Fig. 26. *Thymic carcinoma, epidermoid non-keratinizing.* Edges of the tumour nodule are sharp, with a suggestion of palisading. The cytoplasm is eosinophilic, but there is neither overt keratinization nor intercellular bridges

38

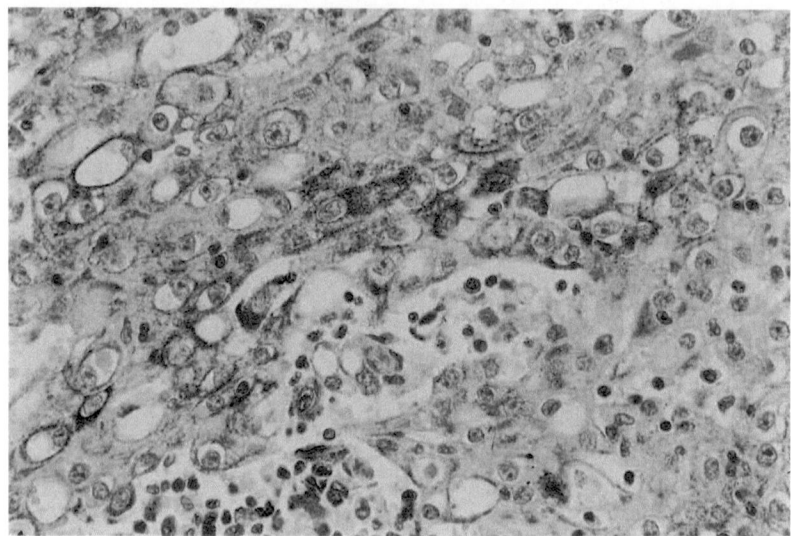

Fig. 27. *Thymic carcinoma, epidermoid non-keratinizing.* Diffuse immunoreactivity for CD5, particularly in some tumour cells located in the centre

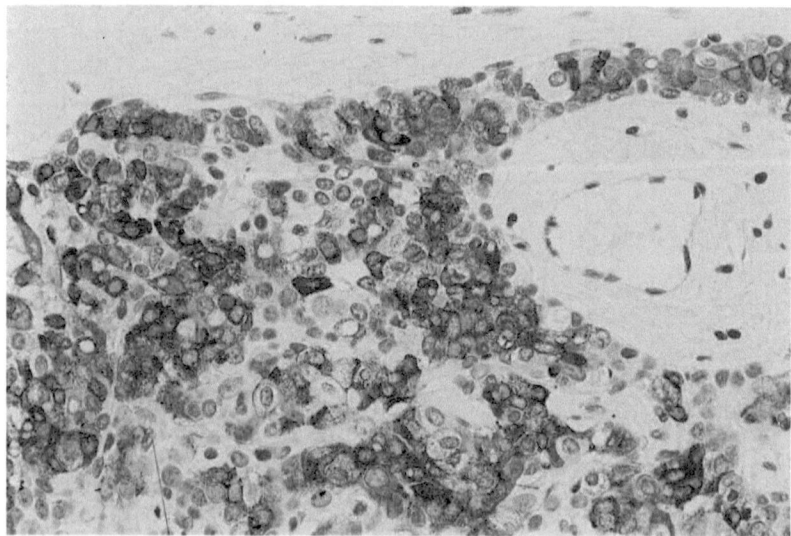

Fig. 28. *Thymic carcinoma, epidermoid non-keratinizing.* Widespread immunoreactivity for synaptophysin

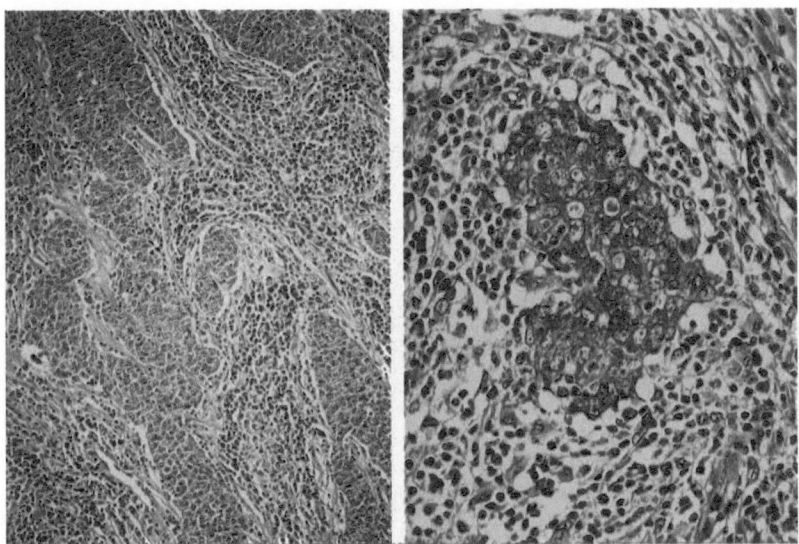

Fig. 29. *Thymic carcinoma, lymphoepithelioma-like.* The low-power view shows tumour nodules separated by wide fibrous bands infiltrated by lymphocytes. The high-power view on the right shows a tumour cluster with a "syncytial" appearance. Lymphocytes are present within and around this tumour nodule

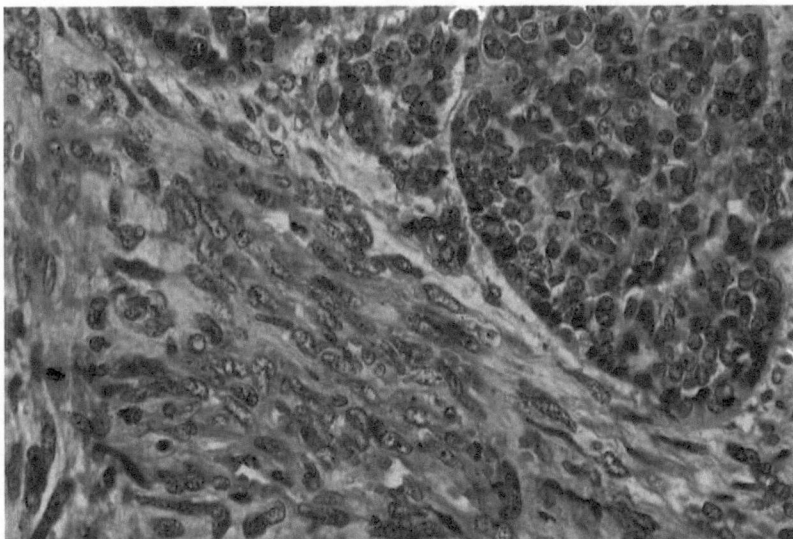

Fig. 30. *Thymic carcinoma, sarcomatoid (carcinosarcoma).* Sharply-outlined areas with a carcinomatous appearance in the upper right alternate with foci having a spindle configuration resulting in a sarcoma-like appearance

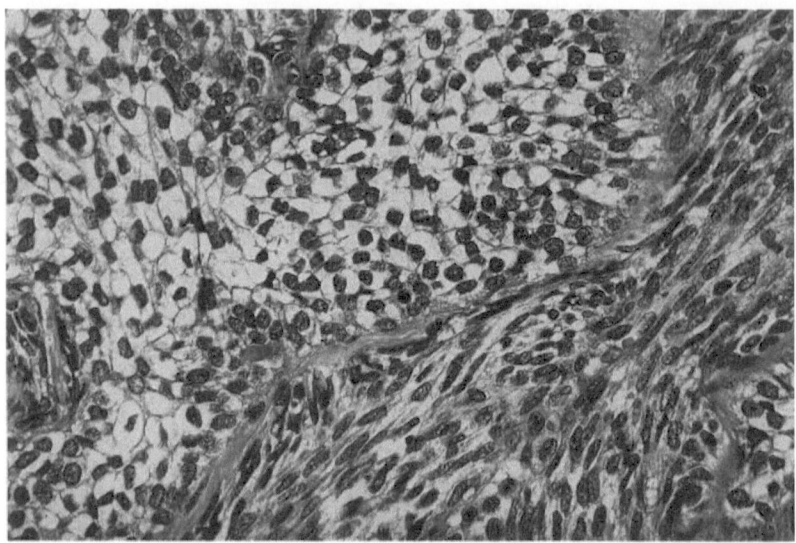

Fig. 31. *Thymic carcinoma, sarcomatoid (carcinosarcoma).* In this particular instance, the carcinomatous component of the tumour has a clear cell appearance

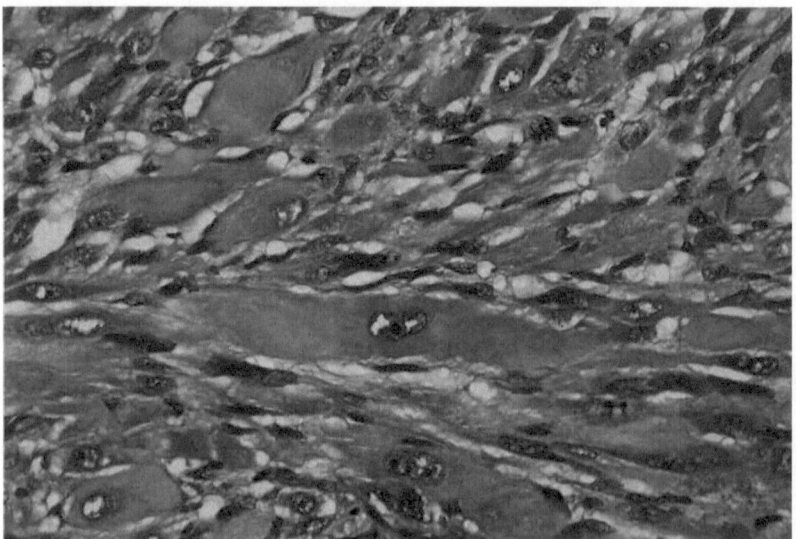

Fig. 32. *Thymic carcinoma, sarcomatoid (carcinosarcoma).* High-power view of the sarcomatoid component exhibiting features suggesting skeletal muscle differentiation

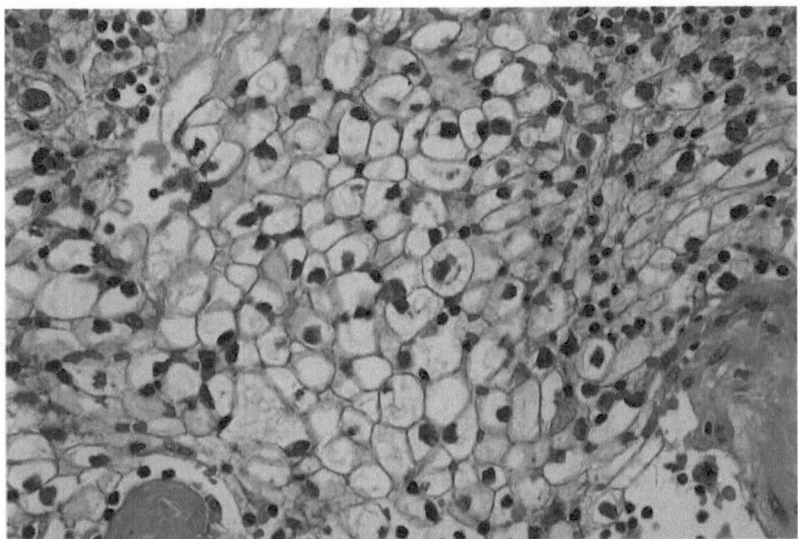

Fig. 33. *Thymic carcinoma, clear-cell type.* The cells have abundant, optically-clear cytoplasm and well-defined cell membranes

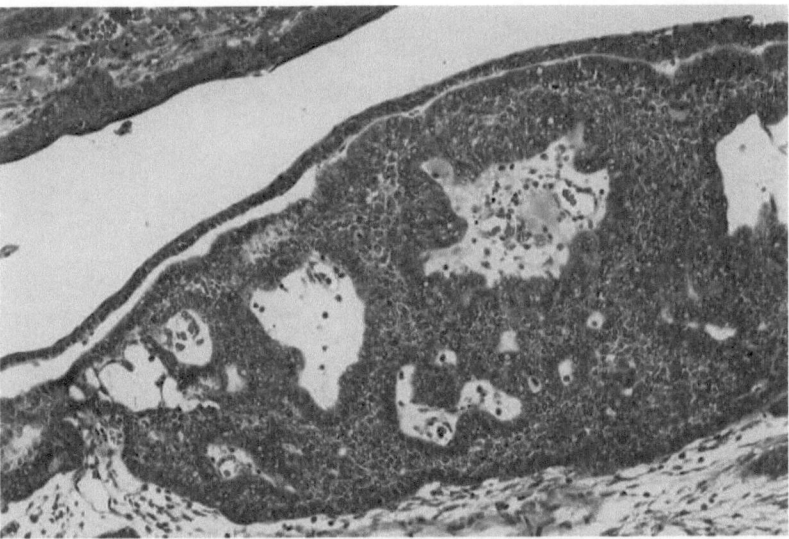

Fig. 34. *Thymic carcinoma, basaloid.* Sharply outlined islands of tumour cells exhibiting a basophilic staining pattern and peripheral palisading are beneath a cystic formation lined by similar cells

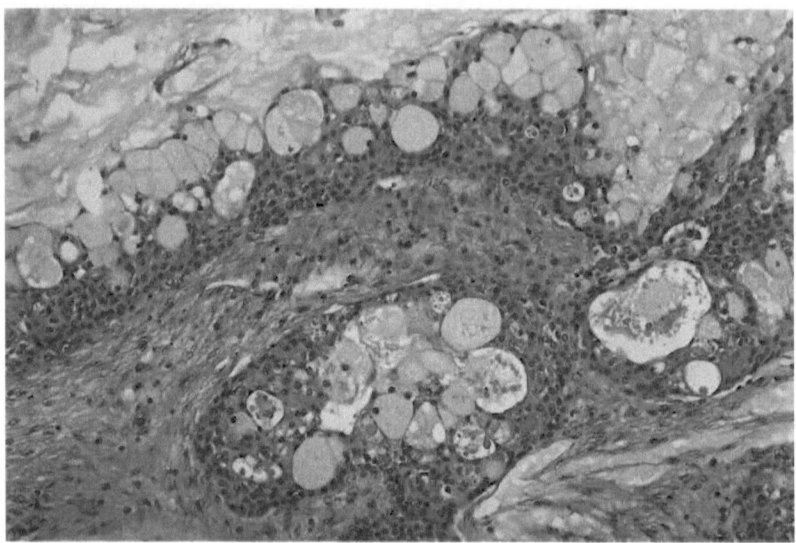

Fig. 35. *Thymic carcinoma, mucoepidermoid type.* Admixture of mucin-producing and squamous cells in a predominantly cystic neoplasm

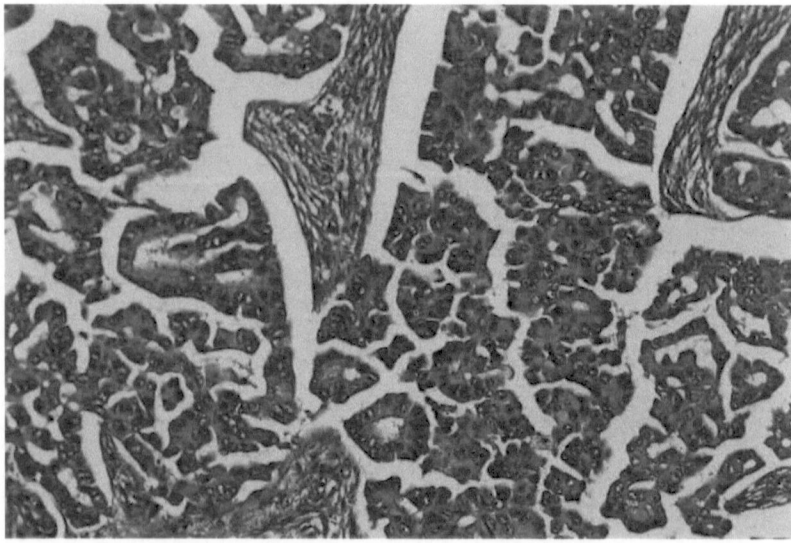

Fig. 36. *Thymic carcinoma, papillary type.* Highly papilliferous configuration resembles papillary carcinoma of the thyroid

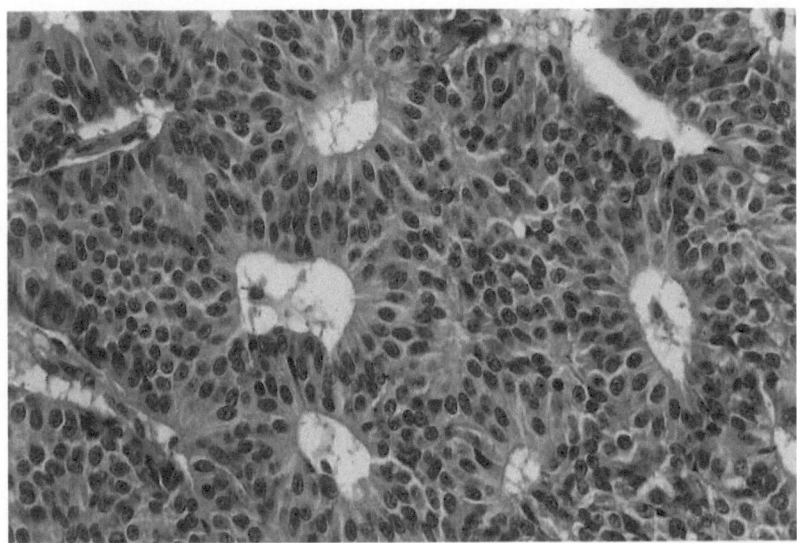

Fig. 37. *Classic carcinoid.* Rosette-like glandular formations with central lumen

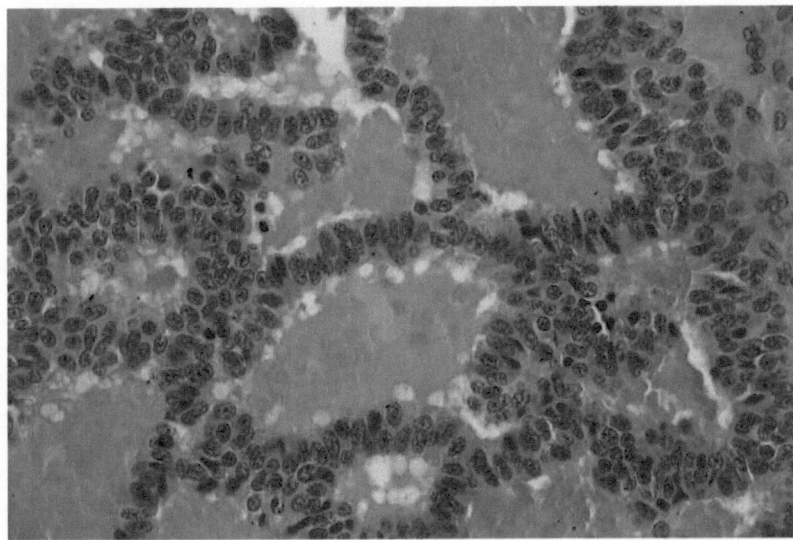

Fig. 38. *Classic carcinoid.* Ribbons and festoons, little atypia, no mitotic activity and no necrosis

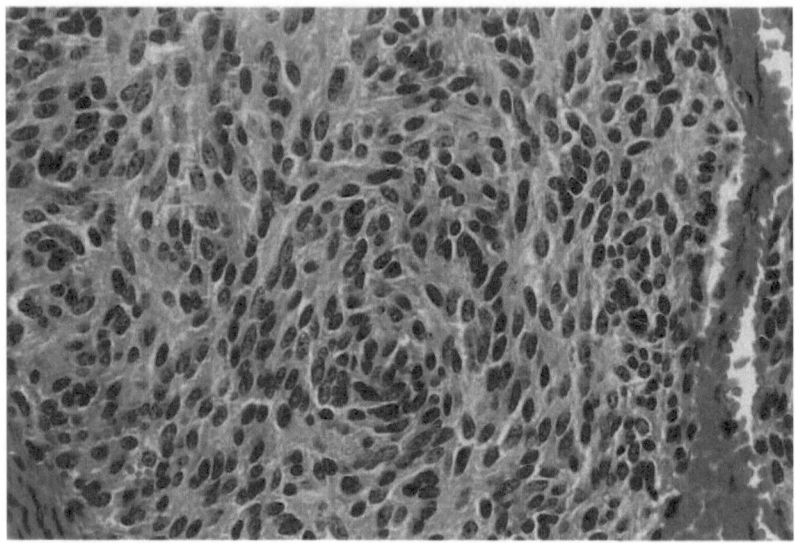

Fig. 39. *Spindle cell carcinoid.* Cells are spindle-shaped and have a vaguely whorling pattern. This tumour needs to be distinguished from type A thymoma

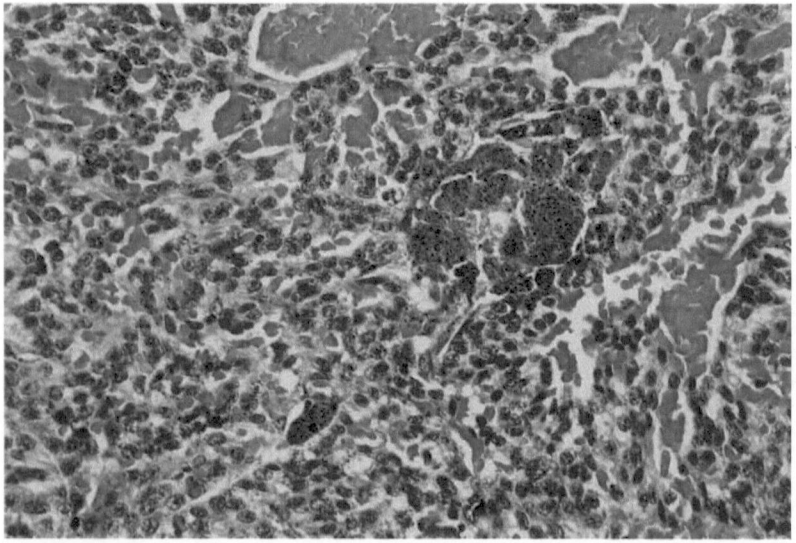

Fig. 40. *Pigmented carcinoid.* Abundant melanin is present in the cytoplasm of some tumour cells

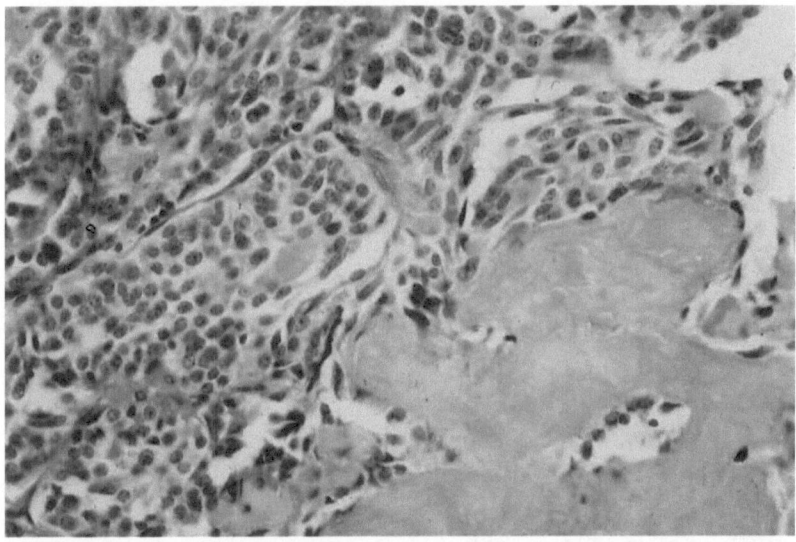

Fig. 41. *Well-differentiated neuroendocrine carcinoma with amyloid (extra-thyroidal medullary carcinoma)*. The tumour cells, which are round to oval, are accompanied by abundant deposition of extracellular amyloid

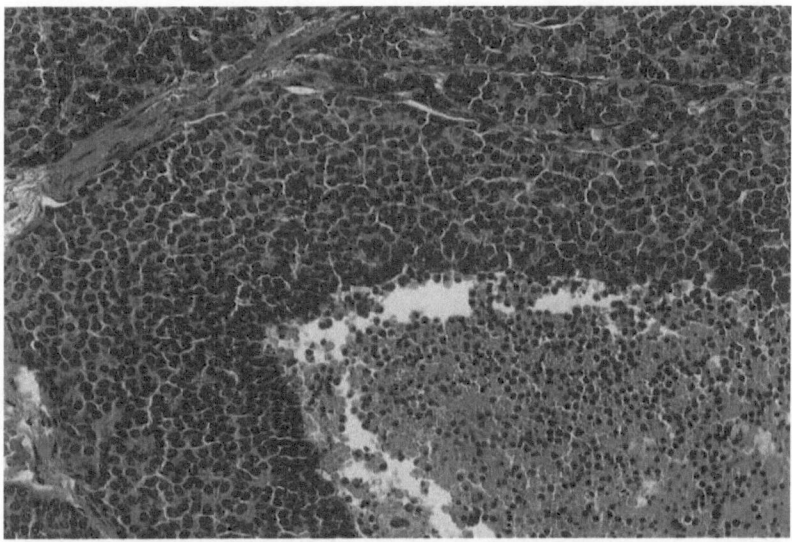

Fig. 42. *Atypical carcinoid*. There is extensive necrosis in the centre of the tumour nest. On high power examination, mitotic features were identified

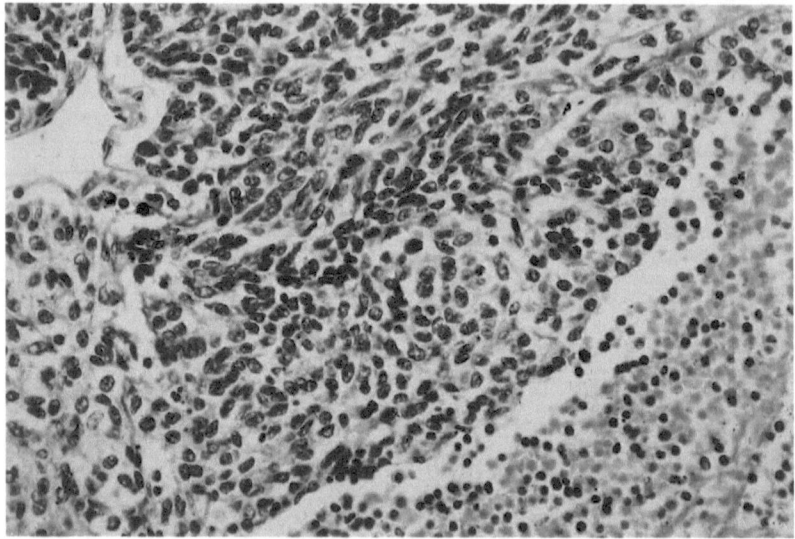

Fig. 43. *Small cell carcinoma.* Small cells with darkly hyperchromatic nuclei and scanty cytoplasm are accompanied by extensive foci of necrosis

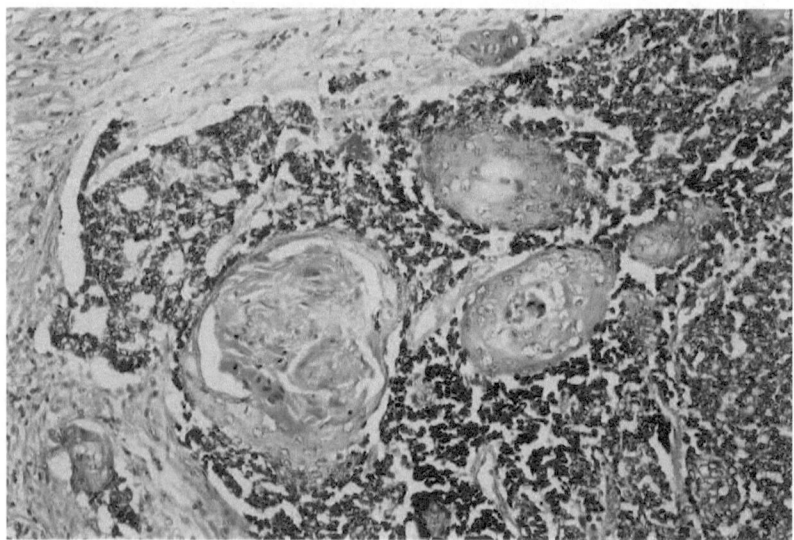

Fig. 44. *Mixed small cell-epidermoid keratinizing carcinoma.* Sharp segregation between foci of small cell carcinoma and the round clusters of keratinizing squamous cells

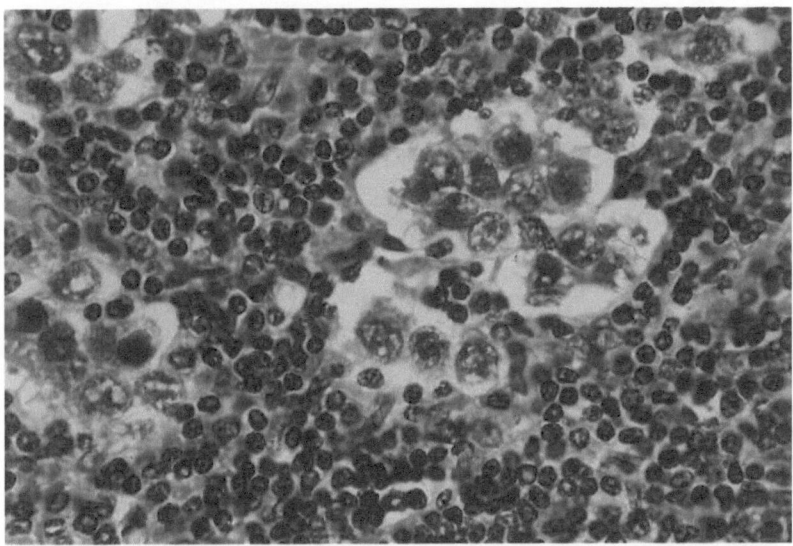

Fig. 45. *Seminoma (germinoma) of the thymus.* Clusters of tumour cells with large nuclei and irregularly shaped prominent nuclei separated by fibrous strands containing abundant lymphocytes and other inflammatory cells

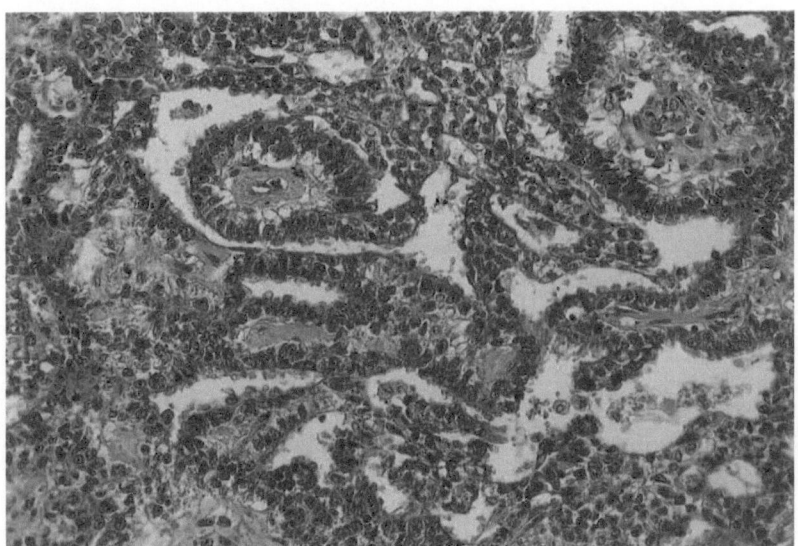

Fig. 46. *Yolk sac tumour.* Pseudo-papillary pattern formed as a result of the development of so-called Schiller-Duval bodies by the tumour cells

48

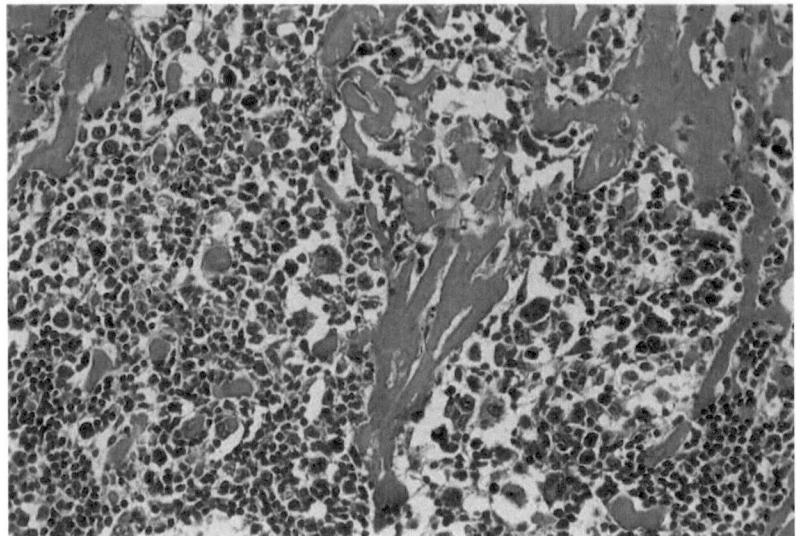

Fig. 47. *Hodgkin lymphoma of the thymus.* Nodular sclerosis type

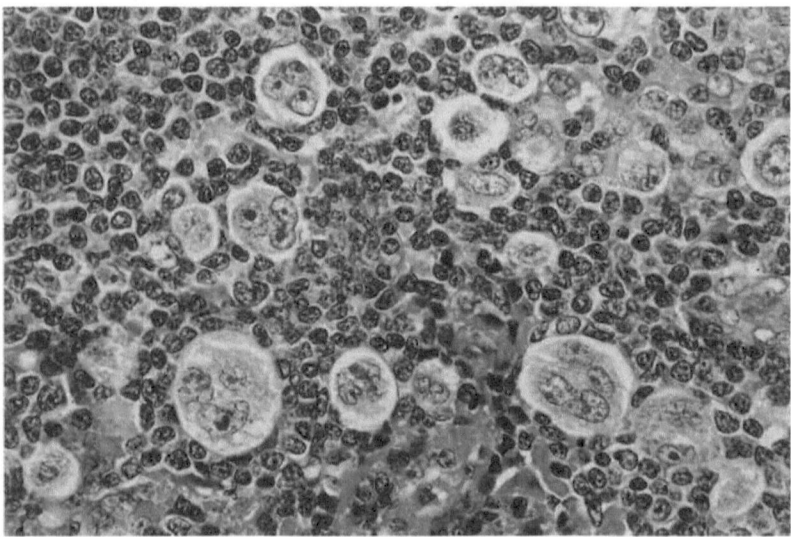

Fig. 48. *Hodgkin lymphoma of the thymus.* Numerous lacunar cells, some of which fulfill the criteria for Reed-Sternberg cells

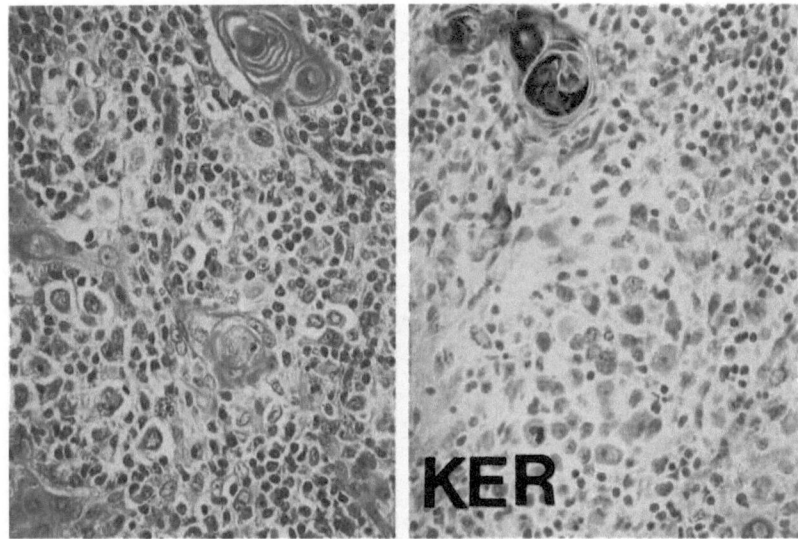

Fig. 49. *Hodgkin lymphoma of the thymus.* Hyperplasia of the entrapped thymic epithelium (highlighted by the keratin stain on the right), may lead to a mistaken diagnosis of thymic carcinoma

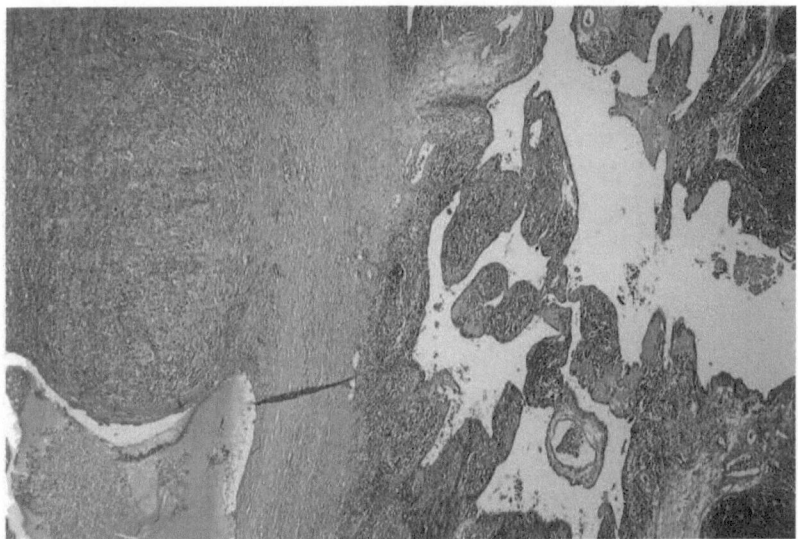

Fig. 50. *Hodgkin lymphoma of the thymus.* The tumour (represented by the solid mass on the *left half* of the photograph) is accompanied by multi-locular thymic cystic formation (*right half*)

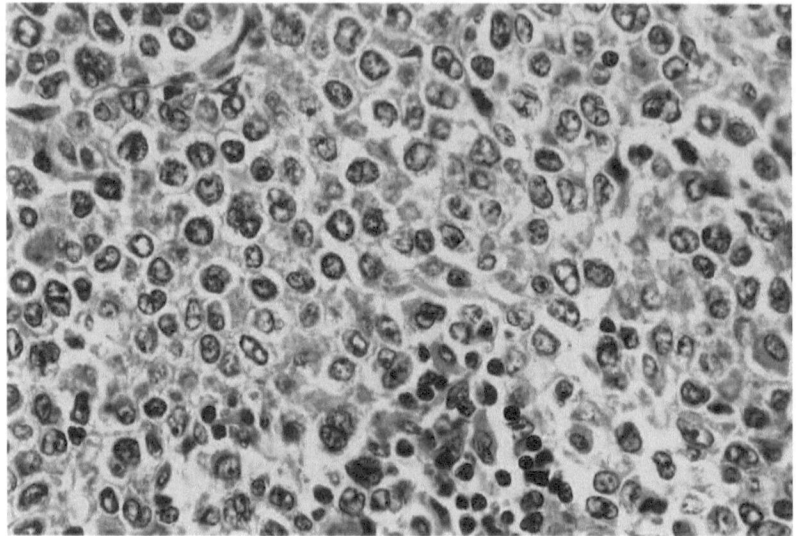

Fig. 51. *Large cell lymphoma of the thymus.* The pattern of growth is diffuse and the nuclei show marked irregularities of the membrane. A few scattered non-neoplastic lymphocytes are present

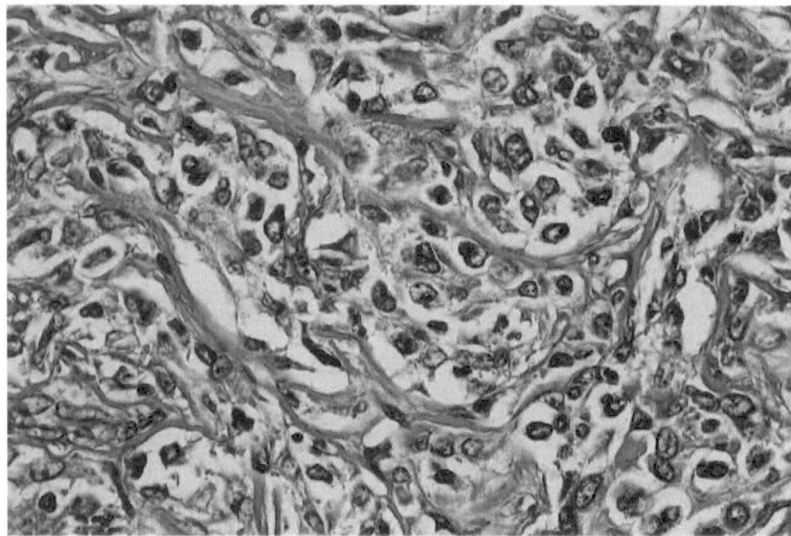

Fig. 52. *Large cell lymphoma with sclerosis of the thymus.* Fibrohyaline bands incompletely divide the tumour cells into nests

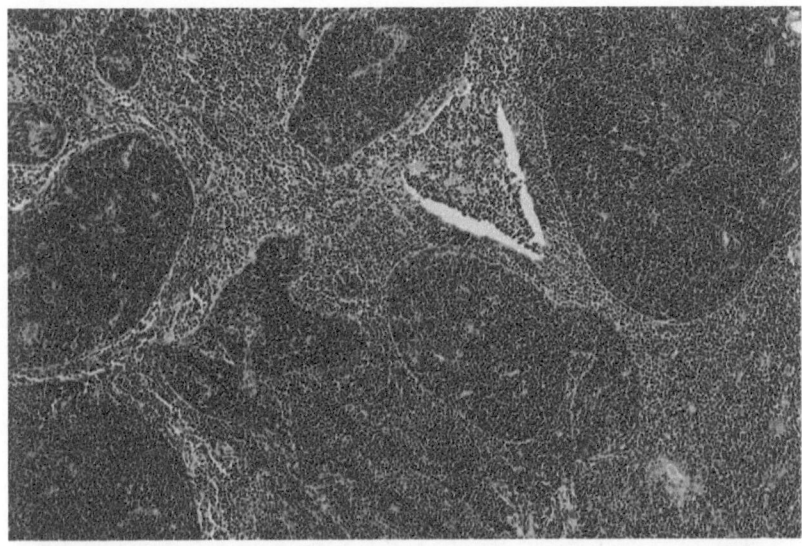

Fig. 53 *Lymphoblastic lymphoma of thymus.* Tumour cells are present both within and between the thymic lobules, which are markedly expanded and deformed

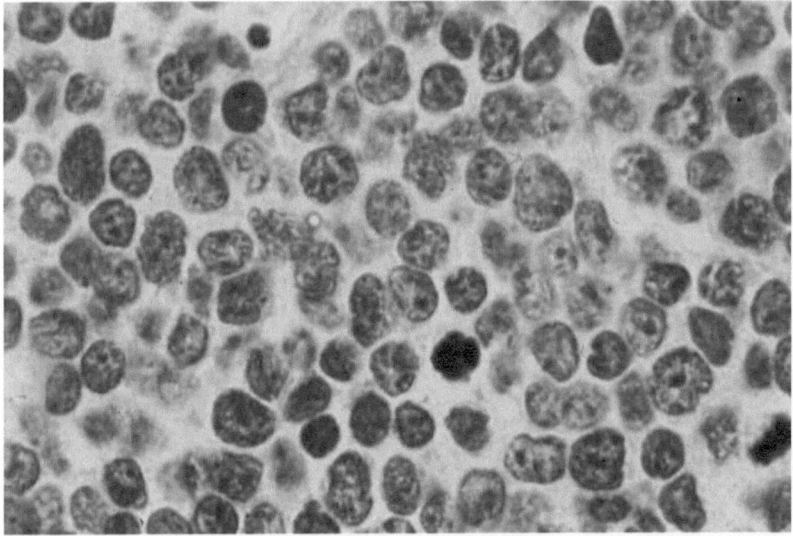

Fig. 54. *Lymphoblastic lymphoma of thymus.* High-power view highlights the high mitotic activity and the convolutions of the nuclear membrane

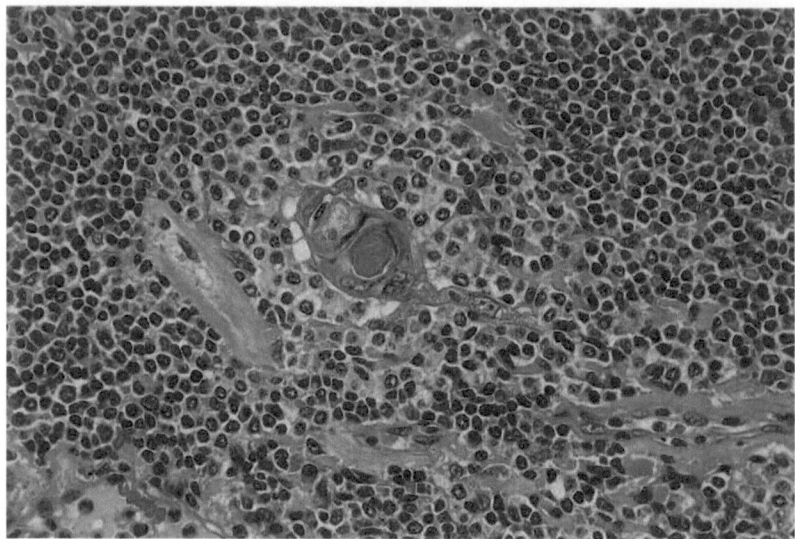

Fig. 55. *Mucosa-associated lymphoid tissue (MALT)-type lymphoma of the thymus.* The small tumour cells surround a Hassall corpuscle and are in turn surrounded by non-neoplastic lymphocytes

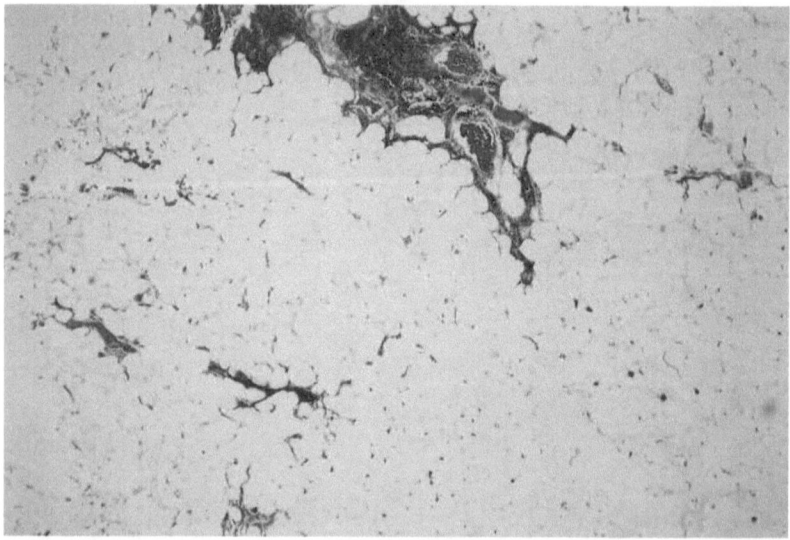

Fig. 56. *Thymolipoma.* Islands of histologically normal thymic tissue in a sea of mature adipose tissue

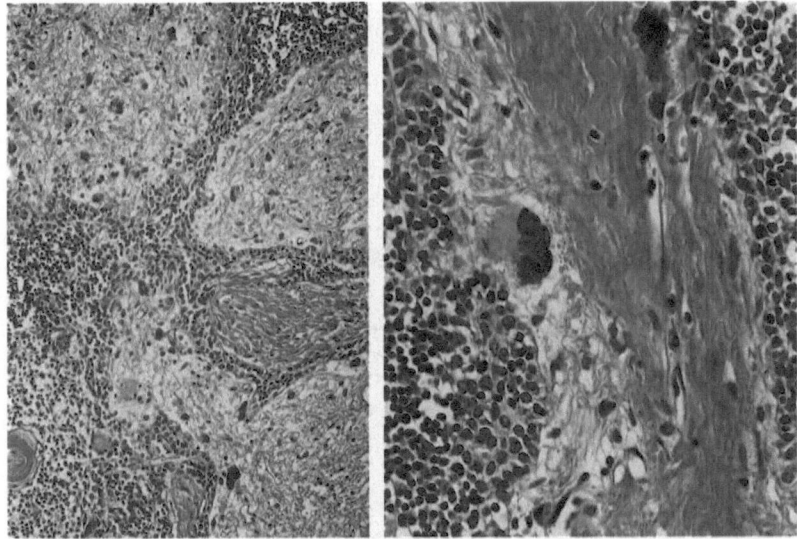

Fig. 57. *Thymoliposarcoma.* A tumour with the microscopic features of the sclerosing form of well-differentiated liposarcoma (atypical lipomatous tumour) involves the thymic stroma. The high-power view on the right shows several bizarre tumour cells

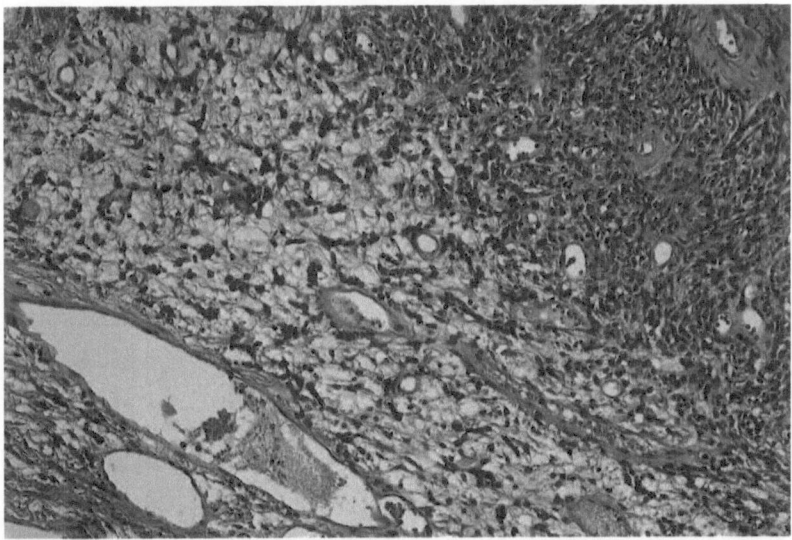

Fig. 58. *Solitary fibrous tumour involving the thymus.* Alternation of hyper- and hypocellular foci and the hemangiopericytoma-like areas characterise this entity

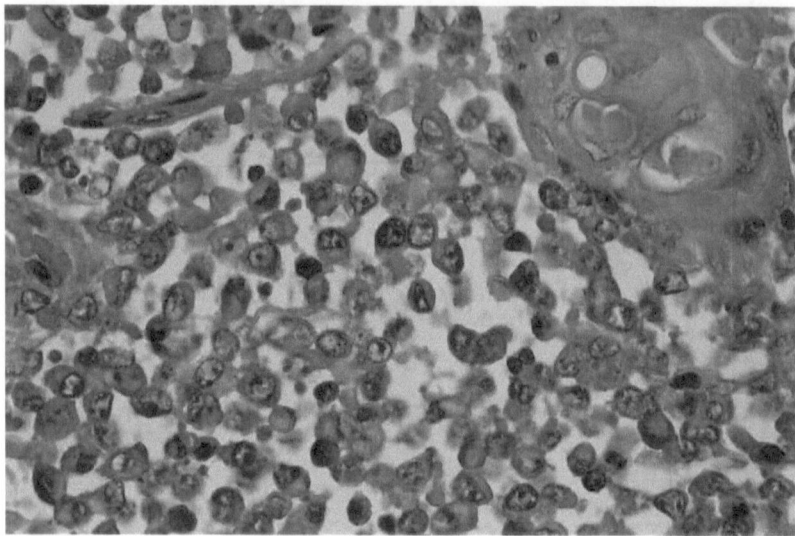

Fig. 59. *Rhabdoid tumour of the thymus.* Oval tumour cells with cytoplasmic homogeneous hyaline "inclusions" that displace the nucleus laterally. A residual Hassall corpuscle at *right upper corner*

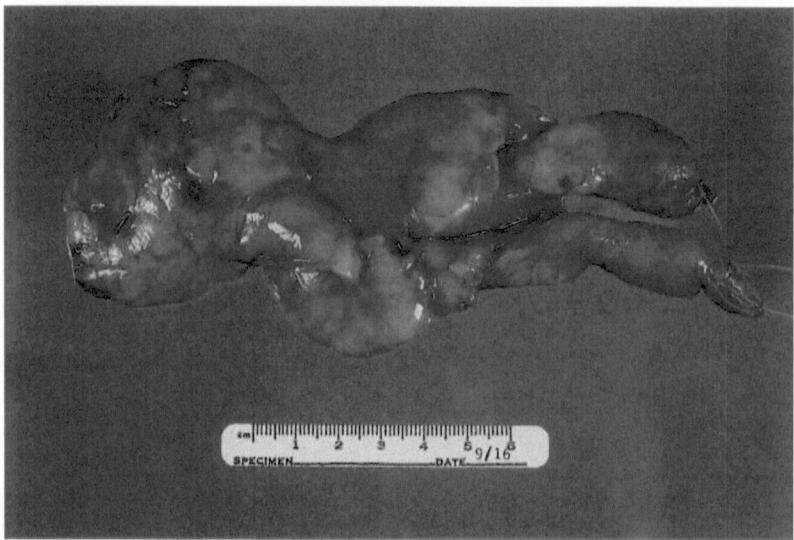

Fig. 60. *True thymic hyperplasia.* This thymus weighed 70 g and was excised from a 26-year-old female. It was microscopically normal, but its weight was beyond the upper limits of normal for this age group (approximately 45 g according to Hammar's table)

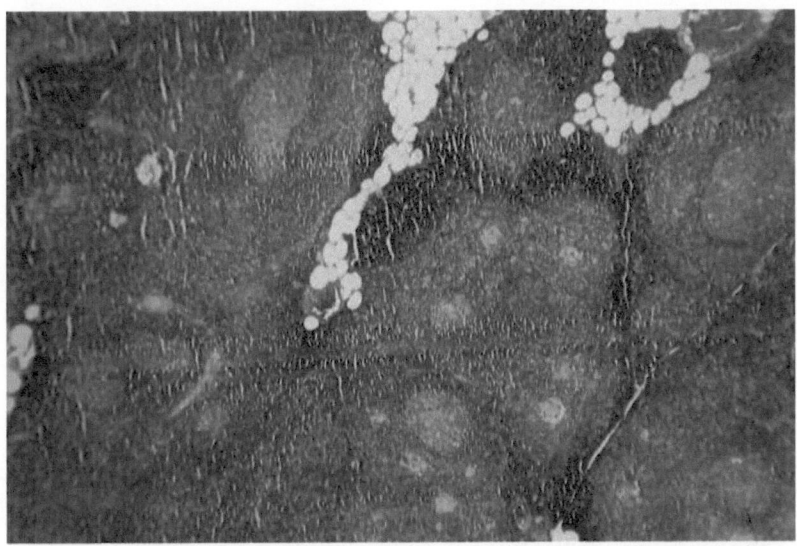

Fig. 61. *Lymphoid hyperplasia of the thymus*. This lesion, which occurred in a patient with myasthenia gravis, shows numerous lymphoid follicles with germinal centres throughout the thymus

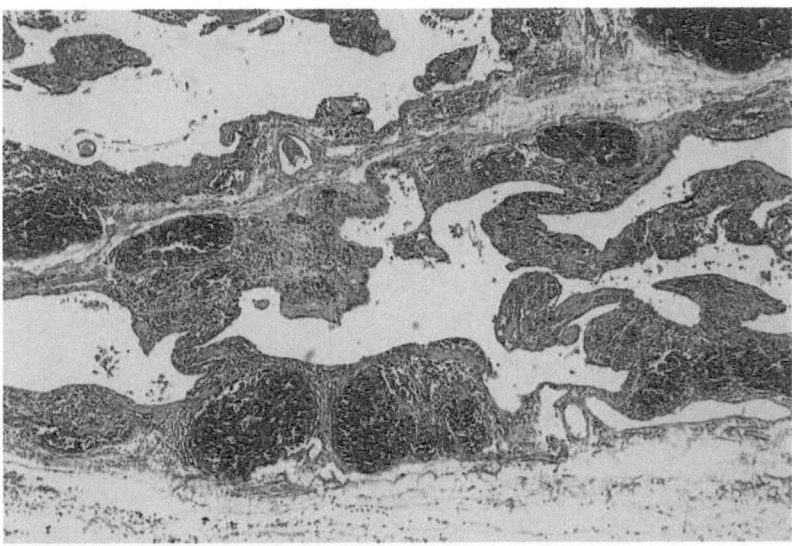

Fig. 62. *Multilocular thymic cyst*. Numerous cystic spaces lined by thymic epithelial cells are separated by septa containing inflammatory cells, some of them in the form of lymphoid follicles

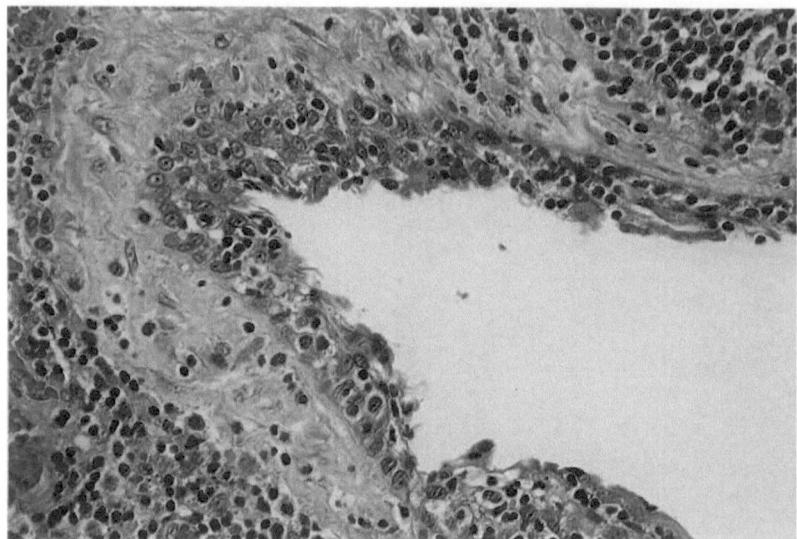

Fig. 63. *Multilocular thymic cyst.* On high-power, the lining of the cyst is of stratified squamous type and infiltrated by the lymphocytes

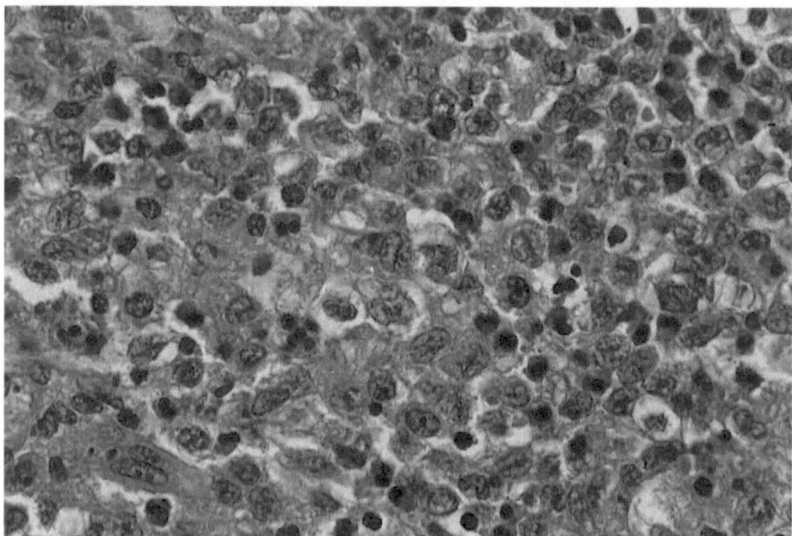

Fig. 64. *Langerhans cell histiocytosis of the thymus.* The Langerhans cells, some of which show nuclear grooves, are admixed with eosinophils and lymphocytes

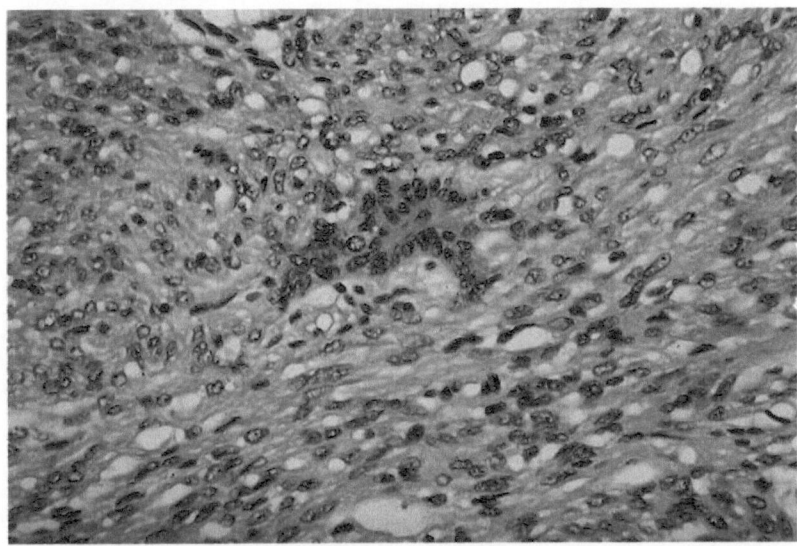

Fig. 65. *Ectopic hamartomatous thymoma.* A cell cluster with a clear-cut epithelial appearance in the centre of the photograph is surrounded by tumour cells having a mesenchymal-like spindle configuration

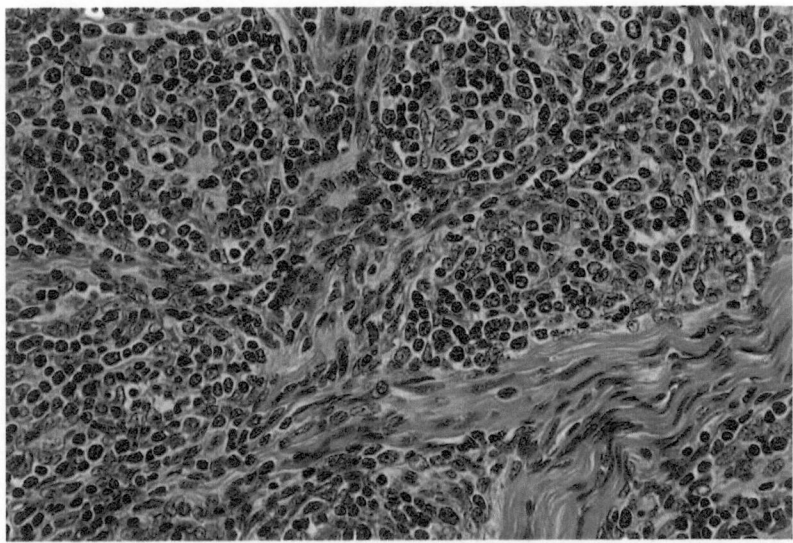

Fig. 66. *Ectopic cervical thymoma.* This tumour corresponds to a type AB thymoma in that it combines lymphocyte-rich areas with spindle cells arranged as bundles

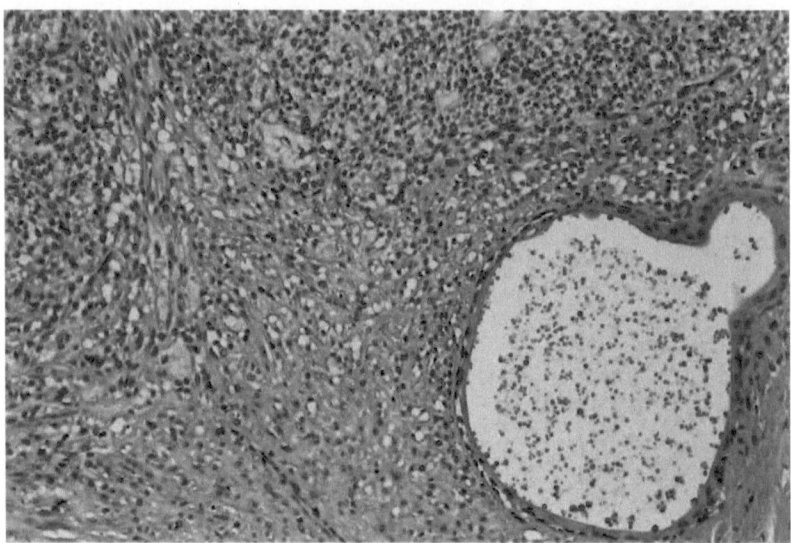

Fig. 67. *Spindle epithelial tumour with thymus-like differentiation (SETTLE).* A large cystic formation containing mucinous material in what is an otherwise solid and rather cellular neoplasm

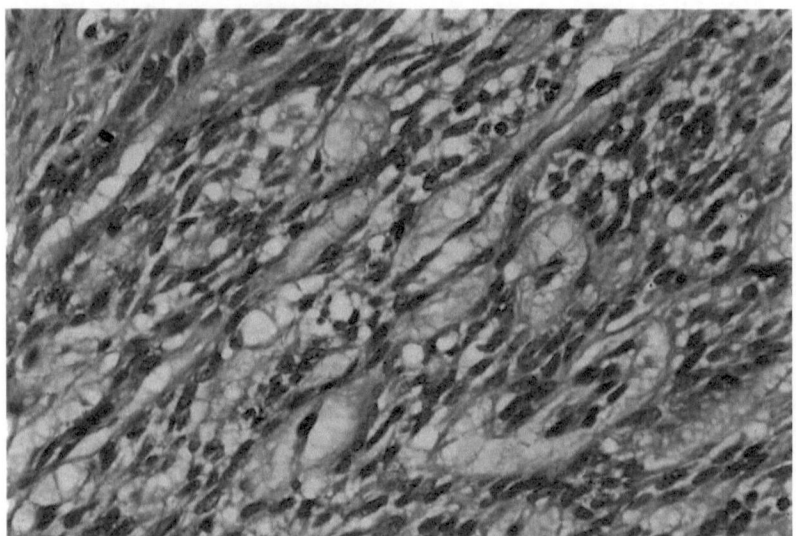

Fig. 68. *Spindle epithelial tumour with thymus-like differentiation (SETTLE).* On high-power, the spindle cells are focally separated by the accumulation of an extracellular mucinous material

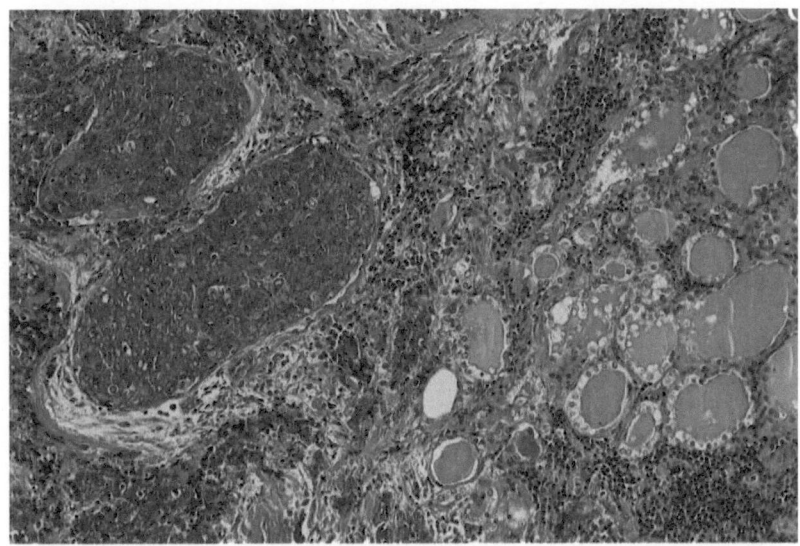

Fig. 69. *Carcinoma showing thymus-like differentiation (CASTLE).* Sharply-outlined foci of tumour infiltrating normal thyroid follicles

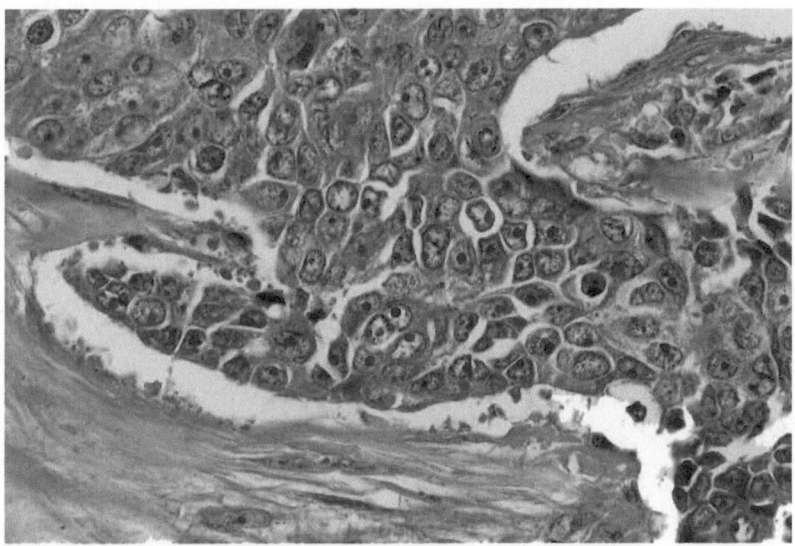

Fig. 70. *Carcinoma showing thymus-like differentiation (CASTLE).* On high-power, the appearance is similar to that of thymic carcinoma of the epidermoid non-keratinizing type

Subject Index